TABLE OF CONTENT

Detox

INTRODUCTION

Detoxification is what your body does naturally to neutralize, transform or get rid of unwanted materials or toxins. It is a primary function of the body, constantly working and interacting with all other functions of the body. So when I am talking about detoxification, it is about improving and optimizing the function of your body's own detoxification systems. This is done by decreasing the amount of toxins we put into our bodies while at the same time supporting our body's detoxification and elimination systems with the nutrients it needs to function properly.

As a culture we are very aware of our external cleanliness. We clean our teeth daily, we bath and wash our hair daily or every other day and we like to look and smell clean because it makes us feel better. Similarly, I see detoxification as internal cleansing. The problem is that it's often hard to know when our internal cleansing mechanisms are not functioning well. Unlike other parts of our body it is very hard to know how well our liver is working, and our liver is the main detoxification organ. Apart from synthesizing and secreting bile, the liver acts as a filter for toxins and bacteria in the blood and chemically neutralizes toxins, converting them into substances that can be eliminated by the kidneys.

Although it is mostly ignored by our current medical system, the detoxification system is a key component of our body's functioning. Most of the molecules made by our bodies every day, are for getting rid of waste products. We need hundreds of enzymes, vitamins and other molecules to help rid the body of unwanted waste products and chemicals. We need to manufacture these molecules to help take the good from what we ingest and get rid of the unwanted. Although the bulk of the work is done by the liver and the intestinal tract, the kidneys, lungs, lymphatic system and skin are all involved in this complex detoxification system.

The purpose of a detoxification program is primarily to support these organs of elimination so that toxins present in the body can be metabolized and excreted. Time and time again I've seen the benefits a good internal cleanse can bring.

We live in a polluted and stressful world. A person's body can become overburdened and strained by contaminants. This contamination can lead to health problems. There are several types of toxins.

- Anti-nutrients such as high fructose corn syrup, trans-fats, caffeine, alcohol, and processed foods
- By-products from the chemical processes that keep us alive such as nitrogen, carbon dioxide, bile, urea, and stool
- Medications used improperly, inappropriately, or too often
- Heavy metals such as mercury, arsenic, lead, cadmium, tin, and aluminum
- Chemicals such as pesticides, herbicides, cleaning products, solvents, and glues
- Allergens such as food, mold, dust, pollen, and chemicals
- Causes of infections such as bacteria, viruses, yeast, and parasites

Further, there are social, emotional, and spiritual challenges that affect health and well-being:

- Stress such as lack of personal time, too much work, excessive worry, too little rest, and financial strain
- Unhealthy mental states such as addictions, overeating, and destructive mental patterns
- Distractions that surround us such as constant noises, smells, lights, and images
- Over-stimulation from advertisements, radio, computers, TV, phones, and pagers
- Lack of spiritual connection, a loss of meaning and purpose
- Isolation, the lack of social support and community
- Nature deprivation, being disconnected from natural environments
- Negative emotions and persistent self-defeating thoughts such as anger, fear, guilt, hopelessness

Detoxification Organs

Our bodies and minds already have the ability to handle these challenges. This process of maintaining physical and emotional balance is called homeostasis. The major body systems that work together to maintain health and balance include our:

- Liver and gallbladder
- Kidneys
- Digestive system
- Skin
- Lungs
- Blood and lymphatic's
- Brain

Our body handles toxins by neutralizing, transforming, or eliminating them. The liver helps transform many toxic substances into harmless agents, while the blood carries waste to the kidneys; the liver also dumps waste through the bile into the intestines, where much of it is eliminated. We also clear toxins when our body sweats. Our sinuses and skin may also be accessory elimination organs, whereby excess mucus or toxins can be released.

Detoxification is the process of clearing toxins from the body by neutralizing or transforming them and clearing excess mucus and congestion. Detoxification also involves dietary and lifestyle changes that reduce intake of toxins and improve elimination. Avoidance of chemicals (from food or other sources), refined food, sugar, caffeine, alcohol, tobacco, and many drugs help to minimize the toxin load. Almost everyone needs to detoxify. We detoxify to clear symptoms, treat disease, and prevent further problems. We also detoxify to rest our overloaded organs of digestion. With a regular balanced diet, devoid of excesses, a less intense detoxification will be indicated. However, when we eat a congesting diet higher in fats, meats, dairy products, refined foods, and chemicals, detoxification becomes more necessary. Who needs to detoxify is based on individual lifestyle and symptoms of toxicity. Common toxicity symptoms include: headache, fatigue, mucus problems, aches and pains, digestive problems, "allergy" symptoms, and sensitivity to environmental agents such as chemicals, perfumes, and synthetics.

Why we need detoxification??

There are no exact symptoms to suggest that your body's natural detoxification system is not working well. Your body may have a problem with detoxification if you have a number of the following symptoms and a clinician has seen you to determine that they are not caused by other medical conditions:

- Fatigue with sleep disruption and brain fog
- Mood disturbance, especially depression, anxiety, fear, and anger
- Muscle aches and joint pain
- Sinus congestion, dark circles under the eyes, and post-nasal drip
- Headaches with neck and shoulder pain
- Bloating and gas
- Irritable bowel, foul-smelling stools, and dark urine
- Weight changes and loss of muscle tone
- Heartburn, recurrent colds, and persistent infections
- Infertility and low interest in sex
- Premature aging and weakness
- Fluid retention and excess weight
- Rashes and canker sores
- Bad breath and body odor

What detoxifications do??

Basically, detoxification means cleaning the blood. This is done by removing impurities from the blood in the liver, where toxins are processed for elimination. The body also eliminates toxins through the kidneys, intestines, lungs, lymph and skin.

A detox program can help the body's natural cleansing process by:

1. Resting the organs through fasting;
2. <u>Stimulating the liver</u> to drive toxins from the body;
3. Promoting elimination through the intestines, kidneys and skin;
4. <u>Improving circulation of the blood</u>; and
5. Refueling the body with healthy nutrients.

Many of the symptoms of a detox are related and build off of each other. You may feel sluggish and hungry all of the time but not have any of the other symptoms. Typically the way you feel is directly related to what you've been eating. If you've ever lost control of your healthy lifestyle and binged on crappy food, you may have felt awful afterward. This feeling can be attributed to the significant toxin buildup in your system.

Detox programs help to "flush" these toxins out of your system using all natural ingredients and plenty of water. By putting only natural foods into your system, your digestive system has a chance to "reset" and use less energy. This gives your body more energy and stability to help enhance sleep, alertness, functional energy, and provide strength for your immune system, which improves hair, skin, and overall health quality.

The Importance of the Colon

The colon is the most important part of your digestive system. In it, there can be years of toxic buildup inhibiting your body from experiencing its most healthy state. A detox works to push this colonic buildup out of your system by flushing it with plenty of fiber and water, cleansing your body and ridding it of the toxins and chemicals you've consumed over your lifetime.

Once this elimination part of the program is over, many detox participants experience weight loss, water weight loss, and a reduction in cravings for salty and sugary foods. Since you've abstained from these foods through the duration of your detox, your body no longer believes these ingredients to be necessary.

Who Shouldn't Try a Detox Diet?

Anyone considering a detox diet should consult a qualified health professional and/or their medical doctor first. Pregnant or nursing women or children shouldn't go on a detox diet. People with certain health conditions such as liver or kidney disease should only try it under the supervision of their primary care provider. It is not intended for alcohol or drug detoxification.

Fatigue, indigestion, cough, muscle pain, and poor sleep can be signs of serious illness. That's why it's important to see a primary care provider for a thorough assessment to ensure that any symptoms are not caused by a medical condition that requires immediate treatment.

Side Effects

One of the most common side effects is headache within the first few days of starting the detox diet, often due to caffeine withdrawal. For this reason, practitioners often suggest gradually decreasing the amount of caffeine prior to starting a detox diet. In addition, some people opt to take time off work to begin a detox diet or start the diet on the weekend.

Other side effects include excessive diarrhea, which can lead to dehydration and electrolyte loss. Constipation may occur if people consume excess fiber without also increasing their fluid intake. Other side effects can include tiredness, irritability, acne, weight loss, and hunger. Any worsening of symptoms or new symptoms that occur during a detox diet should prompt a visit to a qualified health professional.

What should we look for?

It is a good general rule that if you intend to cleanse, and you want to do it a nutritional, safe, healthy way, make sure your cleanse program has the following qualities:

1. **Nutrition**. Unless you intend to do a fast, which is completely separate from a nutritional cleanse, you'll want to go with a detox program that values nutrition and contains daily vitamins, protein, fruits and vegetables, and other healthy foods. Many detox programs are simply diet pills that you take in addition to your normal diet (or they're meant to be your ONLY source of nutrition). These are dangerous and do not provide the benefits your body needs to sustain a detox healthfully. Make sure to pick a product that helps you stay full so that you're less likely to cheat and break your detox.

2. **All Natural**. Unfortunately, the regulations concerning what constitutes "all natural" are incredibly vague. Many companies, especially those with products made outside of the United States, claim that their products are all natural but they may still use trace amounts of artificial ingredients. All natural in its most simple form means any product without artificial colors, flavors, sweeteners or preservatives. If it's got citric acid, it's not all natural. If it's sweetened with Splenda, it's not all natural. Basically if you can't pronounce the ingredients, then it's not all natural. If your grandmother wouldn't recognize an ingredient, then it's not all natural. In general, try to use a detox program that only contains REAL ingredients from the earth, not a lab. If a product contains soy, make sure it is non-genetically modified (non-GMO) and the product uses soybeans instead of a soy isolate.

3. **Vegan**. This should go without saying, but animal products, whether meat or dairy, in general, are packed with fat, hormones, chemicals, cholesterol, salt, and other things that contradict weight loss and a healthy detox. One of the biggest benefits of a detox is reduction of bloating. Animals products directly cause bloating since they have salt, fats, and lactose that can fill your stomach with gas. The types of products that are NOT vegan include those with whey protein, eggs, honey, milk, or meat. Also, it's important to support companies that use animal free ingredients since it is more sustainable and better for the environment.

4. **Gluten Free**. Those with Celiac Disease suffer from a gluten allergy, but they aren't the only ones who should avoid gluten. Gluten can raise insulin levels, cause abdominal cramping and water weight gain, and is usually associated with sugary processed simple carbohydrates that contain the very toxins you're trying to get rid of. Make sure to choose a detox program that is <u>gluten free</u>, which means yeast and wheat free.

5. **Stimulant Free.** Products that promote "weight loss" are often caffeine pills masquerading as detox pills. These stimulants increase your heart rate, can lead to insomnia and loss of concentration, and really contradict the purpose of getting your body back to a natural chemical-free state. Another type of stimulant is a laxative. Laxatives are often used in colon cleanse products to help speed up the elimination portion of the detox. Yes, there are natural laxatives that occur in nature like Senna and other stimulants, mostly in the form of herbal laxative tea. These products, however, can cause severe cramping and can be aggressive and disruptive to your normal daily life. If you want to detox in a safe, easy way, avoid laxatives.

6. **Local Ingredients**. If a product has a bunch of ingredients you can't pronounce and most of them are from outside of the United States, be aware that those ingredients 1. are not regulated by as many US agencies as those ingredients made within the USA, 2. had to travel a long way to get to you, which makes the product worse for the environment, 3. does not support the efforts of local farmers and suppliers. If you want to support American businesses, stay local. Many nutritional cleanses are made in Japan or China, while others are made in California, New York, or Florida.

7. **Taste**. There are plenty of <u>detox/cleanse juices</u> and powders out there that use all natural ingredients and unconventional sources of protein like hemp, flax, rice, or nuts. These products can taste like grass or sand. Hey, if that's what you like, then go right ahead! But most of us want to drink something that we can keep down. If you can't stand the taste of a product then you WON'T stick with your detox, so you might as well not try at all. If you want a fruit-based cleanse, make sure to choose one that has actual fruit in the ingredient list, not fruit puree concentrate or fruit *flavors*.

8. **Probiotics**. Probiotics literally mean "for life." As defined by the World Health Organization (WHO), a probiotic is a living microorganism that, when administered in adequate amounts, confers a health benefit on its host. Probiotic live cultures are friendly bacteria that help to regulate and speed up digestion through the intestines and colon. Probiotic cultures,

specifically L. Acidophillus blend, have been linked to better digestive health and stronger immune systems. Probiotics are typically found in yogurt and other cultured dairy products, but are also available in freeze-dried powder form.

9. **Convenience.** There are several <u>detox programs</u> that involve blending smoothies with your own fruit and vegetables. These programs are usually fairly expensive and can be incredibly inconvenient. Make sure to read customer reviews regarding how simple the program was to follow and how easy it is to make the various meals/drinks.

10. **Price.** The truth is, there are good companies and shady companies in this business. The shady ones will typically offer a "free trial" and then bill your credit card ridiculous amounts for subsequent months. Other, more honest businesses, will charge reasonable rates based off of the cost of the product.

The five basic components of any detoxification program should include:

1. Exercise: every day such as yoga and walking (especially in nature)
2. Regular sweating: a sauna, steam room, or hot room yoga class
3. Healthy nutrition: rich in organic fruits and vegetables and filtered water
4. Self-reflection: such as meditation and breathing-focused relaxation
5. Body-work: such as massage and acupuncture.

Simple & Basic Natural Ways to Detox your Body

These are some simple steps and ways which one can incorporate in daily life to detox the body without using any specific diet plans.

1. Replace a meal each day with a detoxifying smoothie:

Though you never want to go to extreme measures where your diet is concerned, there are some ideas that can work wonders. When it comes to naturally cleansing the body a great measure can be to replace one meal a day with a detoxifying smoothie. This isn't extreme and won't cause any harm, but it can be exceptional for getting rid of the substances that your body doesn't need.

It's important not to jump on the bandwagon for the more extreme measures and to opt for a smoothie that uses natural ingredients at the core. Rather than turning to a premade concoction or chemically enhanced smoothie, just turn to natural foods that will get you cleansed properly. This can not only help with weight loss, but also with keeping the digestive system working the way that it should.

Turning to a smoothie for one of your meals is a great way to jumpstart your metabolism and to kick your digestive system into overdrive. You will notice that natural energy that you feel and you will also enjoy that some of the symptoms that you suffer with daily are gone with this natural boost.

2. Turn to organic foods when possible:

While you don't have to eat only organic, there are certain foods where this is a necessity. The food list known as the "Dirty Dozen" contains a list of foods where pesticides and preservatives can build up and therefore be consumed and ingested by you during digestion.

The rule of thumb generally goes that if you eat the peel or the outside of the fruit or vegetable that you should really opt for organic. Strawberries, apples, and tomatoes are good examples of the types of foods where organic really does matter.

When you choose the right organic foods then you avoid the toxins that can be harmful to your health. This is a simple way of detoxifying the body and all it takes is making good choices at the grocery store.

Be diligent about knowing which organic foods really count, reading labels, and staying away from foods that could harm you. Making healthy choices like this will really help you to get rid of toxins that you were previously ingesting, and get your body to a much cleaner and healthier point.

3. Get a good and intense massage:

We tend to think of massage as a relaxing luxury, which of course it can be in some instances. Though massage can certainly be a nice luxury or way of treating yourself, it also happens to be a good way of detoxifying the body as well. It's all in the type that you get and the way that you use this to better your health and your life.

Suffice it to say that if you are interested in getting rid of toxins in the body, you absolutely have to get a good intense massage that focuses greatly on the pressure points within the body. A typical Swedish massage is good, but something more intense and focused like a Sports massage can work even better.

You want to get deep into the muscle tissue to make this work for you. When you push on these pressure points or spots where toxins tend to build up, then you give them a chance to release. This helps you to naturally detox the body and get rid of the things that may have been making you sick.

4. Drink far more water:

Even if you think that you are drinking enough water in a day, take your intake to a whole new level. If there is one thing that can easily and naturally help you to detox your body, it's definitely water. We tend to think that we're drinking enough when we really need to increase our intake dramatically.

Water can help to flush out your system naturally, and if you drink enough if it then this happens routinely. Proper water intake can contribute to clearer skin, properly functioning organs, and a more effective circulatory, respiratory, and digestive system. So this one simple substance can offer great help to our entire body and the way that it functions.

Forget all the rules that you have heard through the years about how much water is enough. Eight glasses in the minimum, so it's time to dramatically increase your intake if you want the best health benefits. Water should be your drink of choice and should be your choice with meals, as well as before and after. You will see some of the health benefits readily and enjoy some of the longer term ones down the line.

5. Replace the morning coffee with green tea:

A little caffeine is okay, but you do want to be careful about how much you take in throughout a day or week. You also want to be careful about where you get your caffeine from and how much you take in at any one time. Though an occasional cup of coffee is fine, if you are after detoxifying the body, then you want to change things up a bit.

Green tea offers important antioxidants that our body needs in the most natural form. It offers a slight caffeine boost that can help to get you jump started n the morning, just as coffee does. So if you choose to replace your morning cup of coffee with a cup of green tea you still get a caffeine boost and some actual health benefits as well.

Learning to detox the body doesn't have to be complicated, but it does mean that you will have to make healthy choices that really work for you. This means that you will have to make some adjustments, but they are well worth it.

If you can lean to embrace green tea as one example you are getting a healthy boost of caffeine that naturally helps with detox and gives you some very important antioxidants you need to stay healthy in the short and long term.

6. Get in more exercise and sweat it out:

We all know that exercise is an essential part of a truly healthy lifestyle and that it helps with weight loss—but there is much more to it than that! When it comes to naturally and effectively cleansing the body, exercise can be a great option to turn to. Though many people don't think of exercise in this manner, it can be what helps you with the cleansing process dramatically.

When you are exercising you are not only helping the body to shed fat and excess weight, but you are also helping to get rid of toxins that may build up. As you sweat these toxins can come out and therefore the cleansing is taking place. Not only that but you are also helping with digestion, circulation, and to keep the organs functioning as they should with a challenging fitness regimen.

The perspiration, the breathing, and the movement all help the body to achieve fitness and also to get rid of the bad and potentially harmful substances that have built up over time.

If you opt to make exercise a regular function in your life, then you can assist the body in the cleansing process on a regular basis. So sweat it out at the gym, not only because it makes you feel good and releases the best hormones, but also because it can help you to naturally cleanse in the process.

7. Eat more fiber in its most natural form:

You've probably heard it time and time again that you need to be eating more fiber in your diet. Not only is this part of a healthy diet that will contribute to weight loss, but it's also an essential way of cleansing the body in its most natural form. Fiber can be an excellent supplement for a variety of reasons, and cleansing is just one of them.

Our bodies, particularly our digestive tracts, tend to hold onto substances that enter after time. This may be toxins, preservatives from foods that we eat, or just waste that is not being properly disposed of by the body. Whatever the cause, the end result is that you may feel bloated, weighed down, unusually tired, and therefore health problems may result out of this.

When you introduce a proper serving of fiber into your diet, it helps to keep the digestive tract working properly. This means that all toxins, excessive waste, and anything else that has built up in the digestive tract will move through rapidly. You feel healthier and your digestive process works in the way that it is intended to.

There are some great fiber supplements out there, but you should try to eat it naturally whenever possible. Fresh fruits and vegetables, beans and legumes, and whole grains are all excellent sources of fiber.

Start slowly to avoid adverse effects, but when you become regular with your bowel movements you will know that cleansing is happening and the body is working in the way that it is intended to.

8. Try fasting for a day or two:

You don't have to go to extreme measures as so many cleansing programs will tell you to do. Simply fasting for a day or two and replacing foods with natural juices made from fresh fruits and vegetables can really help. You don't have to do this often, but you should make it a priority in your life.

When you give your body a chance to rest in this capacity, then it has time to recuperate and rejuvenate. The organs don't have to be focused on digestion and breaking down food and potential toxins. So as they rest they have a chance to recharge, and that means that you are going to come back from this with natural energy and a more effective digestive system.

Perform a fast like this when you have some time at home and can be away from any food temptations. Try do perform this on a weekend where it's much easier for you to fast and to let the body rest and recharge. You will be surprised at how much natural energy you feel and how much better you feel afterwards.

9. Get in more sleep each night:

You may look at sleep as a luxury, but it's an important part of a healthy lifestyle. Without proper sleep you can gain weight, you may have a compromised immune system, and of course you lack natural energy. Sleep deprivation is unfortunately all too common as we put this off in the interest of getting other things done.

The problem is that lack of sleep can catch up on you after awhile. The body wears down and this shows through in a compromised immune system that means you get sick more easily.

You also have a lack of willpower and lack of energy to make healthy choices for yourself when you feel exhausted. You are ultimately not taking care of yourself in the proper way—and that's not good for your health or your ability to naturally cleanse.

When you try to get 7-8 hours of sleep each night you give your body a chance to rest and recuperate. This is not a luxury but an important way that your body rebuilds and prepares for the activities that you have ahead the next day.

It's imperative to rest and take care of yourself in this manner not only to function properly, but to keep the bad and harmful substances out as well.

10. Avoid obvious environmental toxins:

Some toxins are quite obvious in their presence and their ability to make you sick over time—these are the ones to avoid at all costs. When you can feel the presence of substances that may be making you sick or that can show up in an unsavory way later, then you know that these contribute to a buildup of the things that you don't want or need in your system.

Environmental toxins can range from smog and diminished air quality to second hand smoke. Any chemical type of fumes such as those that may come from a factory are never good for you. If something doesn't smell or feel right, then chances are that it's doing absolutely no good to your system either.

If you have the ability to avoid these substances, particularly something like second hand smoke then it's important to do so. This will ensure that you breathe in good clean air and get rid of the toxins that have built up over time. When in doubt, stay away from any environment, fumes, or substances that can work against your ability to naturally cleanse and care for yourself in this important way.

11. Turn to probiotics to get rid of the bad bacteria and welcome in the good kind:

You may have heard of probiotics or perhaps you don't know much, but these powerful substances help to naturally eliminate bad bacteria in the body. Knowing that they work in this way, it's time to put probiotics to work for you.

Here are some things to keep in mind as you turn to probiotics for a natural cleansing process:

- You have probably heard of probiotics in certain foods such as yogurt and they are continuing to grow in popularity.
- In its natural form, probiotics are a natural and good bacteria that help to regulate and balance out the balance of organisms.
- The most notable application for probiotics is in the digestive system where harmful bacteria and other organisms can grow over time.

- You can turn to certain foods for probiotics and you can also find them in supplement form.
- They can be of great help in not only helping to regulate the bacteria that builds up in your intestines, but also in your ability to get rid of these harmful substances once and for all.
- Since the digestive tract is the most obvious area where these substances can build up, probiotics are an obvious and very helpful tool to assist.
- The use of probiotics not only helps you to keep the digestive system working properly, but also work as a cleansing agent.
- If you turn to them regularly then you can expect to have a fully functional digestive system and to ensure that the presence of these good bacteria will keep you from developing any health problems moving forward.

12. Try yoga for a new type of exercise and meditation:

We already know that exercise is good for our health and for our ability to cleanse naturally. Taking it one step further, yoga can be one of the most helpful types of exercise out there when it comes to the body's natural ability to cleanse and get rid of toxins that have built up over time.

Yoga is not only a great form of exercise, but can also help you to meditate as well. So you get rid of stress as you work through the movements. This is good for the body and the mind as you have a chance to recharge.

These flexibility and balance type of movements can be instrumental to your ability to breath in good cleansing oxygen and breathe out harmful substances within the body. As you move through these poses and breathe properly, you are relieving stress and helping the body to cleanse in a very natural and effective way. You are getting deep down into muscle tissue as you would with a massage, and you are also helping to breathe out toxins that have built up in your system over time. This is one example of how cleansing can help the circulatory system in a dynamic way that has many other helpful applications as well.

13. Learn to incorporate superfoods into each meal:

The great thing about superfoods is that they contain important nutrients and antioxidants which our bodies need to fight off infections. The presence of these antioxidants and nutrients in the body help to fight off harmful toxins and substances that may compromise our immune system and our overall health—so the inclusion of them in our diets is critical.

Superfoods are a delicious and nutritious group of foods including foods rich in Omega 3 fatty acids like:

*Salmon
*Tuna
*Avocado
*Walnuts
*Almonds
*Olive   Oil
*Flax Seeds

You can also turn to fruits and vegetables that are bright in color as that means that their dark hue contains plenty of antioxidants. Options such as these make great choices for this reason:

*Blueberries
*Raspberries
*Spinach
*Kale
*Eggplant
*Tomatoes
*Carrots
*Sweet
*Apples

Try to incorporate super foods into every meal and enjoy how beneficial they are. They not only make for healthy and low fat food choices, but they also help you to boost your antioxidant intake.

These substances can help you to not only cleanse and get rid of harmful substances that have built up, but also fight off any harmful agent that may be trying to attach your system. Something as small as a virus or as harmful as a disease is more easily fought off when you include super foods and their important antioxidant concentration.

14. Cut out simple carbohydrates, white sugar and flour, and any fried foods:

The white bread that you probably enjoyed as a kid is doing absolutely nothing for your overall health. The starchy sides at dinner like white rice or pasta are as damaging to your waistline and your health as the more extreme donuts, cakes, and cookies that you enjoy. Many people don't understand just how harmful products made with white sugar or flour can be, but they result in toxins in the body that you don't want. These simple carbohydrates make you feel full and satisfied when you eat them, but behind the scenes you are experiencing a surge and then fall of your blood sugar level. This isn't good for your appetite or your health!

The same dire consequences of simple carbohydrates are a major component of the very toxins that build up in your digestive system. These are not the types of substances or preservatives that you need, and that's why fiber rich whole grains and complex carbohydrates are so vital to your health. They ensure that the digestive system works the way that it is intended to. So as you move towards complex carbohydrates which are better for digestion, you also want to be sure that you get rid of the simple carbohydrates in the process. The rise and fall of blood sugar is not good for weight loss and the deposit of preservatives and harmful substances result in toxins that can slow you down and ultimately make you sick in the process.

15. Learn to properly manage your stress:

What you know is that stress isn't good for you. What you realize is that to properly take care of yourself and practice a truly healthy lifestyle means to properly manage your stress. What you probably don't realize is that if you let stress get the best of you it can mean that your body is not operating at an optimal level.

You are not releasing good hormones when your body feels stress. As a matter of fact your body may result through weight gain, illness, and a complete lack of energy when stress is present. You are more prone to make improper health choices and more likely to feel depressed and ultimately become sick easier.

When you feel stress the body is holding onto the harmful toxins and therefore is slowed down. When you learn to manage stress properly you are taking a good measure at naturally cleansing the body. This is not only a great way to take care of yourself, but to ensure that none of the harmful substances take residence in your body and contribute to improper health in the long run.

16. Turn to home remedies for illness rather than antibiotics:

The very medications that are intended to help your illnesses or health conditions may be contributing to toxins in the body. Though antibiotics and other medications are intended to help you to stay healthy, they also contain harmful substances that can build up in your intestines and digestive system over time.

Though some medications may be very necessary, it's always best to try home remedies whenever possible. If you can fight off a common illness using options like ginger, garlic, a smoothie, or other natural herbs or plants, then you have a good chance at achieving better health and performing a cleanse in the process. The natural home remedies help to get rid of the illness in the way that your body requires. So as they are fighting off the substances or viruses that are making you sick, you are also getting rid of all other harmful toxins in the body. You feel great as you are fighting off illness through natural means and performing a cleanse in the process-and that's good for everything!

17. Increase circulation by massaging pressure points and skin brushing:

You probably brush your hair and your teeth every day, but more than likely you don't stop to think about brushing your skin. The truth is that brushing a fine bristle brush gently over all of your skin surfaces can be an excellent way to stimulate circulation. Here's how it works:

- Fine a fine bristle brush that is gentle not harsh and begin at the feet with the slow and subtle brushing motions.
- Work your way slowly up from the feet to the legs and up the entire body.
- Take the time to really focus on areas that feel tight or that may be prone to circulation issues such as the ankles, knees, and even arms.
- Repeat the motion a couple of times each week to get the maximum benefits.

- While this often looked to as a method to help to eliminate cellulite, the truth is that this is good at stimulating circulation and ridding the body of toxins that may build up over time

Many people don't take the time to focus on circulatory issues, particularly if they are younger. This is not a problem just for the older because circulation is important at any stage of your life. Be careful to ensure that you keep the circulation running in the body at all times and focus on areas where the toxins may tend to gather.

Another way to generate and promote good circulation is of course to focus on pressure points. This will help not only to ease tension as with a massage, but also to keep the circulatory system working the way that it should. As you focus on these pressure points such as the temples, the palms of your hands, the balls of your feet, and so on, you are releasing tension from the body.

You are also helping to gently and effectively release toxins from the body in the process of doing this as well. When you press gently on these pressure points you can feel it almost instantly with the release of tension.

It helps to stimulate your circulation as well and that means that the toxins are pushed to the surface and then flushed out. Be sure that as with massage of any type that you are drinking plenty of water to help flush out the toxins naturally. Partnering skin brushing with focus on the pressure points can be quite helpful with pushing the toxins out of the body and releasing any build up tension as well.

18. Promote elimination through proper diet and hydration:

The truth is that most of us don't properly eliminate each and every day. Unless you are very regular with your bowel movements and even your urination, you are holding onto waste in the body that need not be there. So this is where you must really focus some concerted effort on elimination, and put major emphasis on the diet that you keep and how hydrated you are.

Start by taking a long hard look at your diet and then work your way out from there:

-Are you eating enough fiber each day?
-Are you eating the right foods such as fresh fruits and vegetables, lean proteins, beans and legumes, whole grains, good fats, and low fat dairy?
-How much water do you realistically drink in a day?
-Do you find yourself feeling unusually thirsty at any point?
-How often do you urinate throughout the day?
-How often do you have bowel movements?

Believe it or not, these are all important questions for your health and for learning to naturally and effectively cleanse. If you are dehydrated that's not good for your overall health. Not only that but it also means that you are not getting enough water to flush out your digestive system properly and move the toxins out.

If you aren't eating enough fiber or a mix of the right foods, then you simply aren't evacuating enough. If you don't have enough bowel movements, that waste material can end up being stored by the body and the end result is that it turns into toxins. This is nothing that you may want to think about, but it can contribute to an unhealthy and improperly working system in the body.

19. Eliminate common sources of toxins such as excessive caffeine, alcohol, tobacco, and processed foods:

The very things that you turn to for bad habits or use to help relax you can be contributing to your inability to cleanse. These substances or bad habits translate directly or indirectly to toxins in the body. The end result is that they keep you from being healthy and may actually make you sick.

The most obvious is tobacco in any form, but of course smoking being the most common type. Smoking offers only harmful substances into your body such as nicotine, which of course can contribute to long term health problems.

You might not realize it, but excessive alcohol or caffeine can act much in the same way. Having a bit of caffeine or alcohol isn't the problem, but when you binge or drink too much of either, it's not a good thing. Over time these can turn into toxins that the body can't process. You will feel the dependence and the health problems will keep mounting.

The same goes for processed foods, fried foods, or others that are made with unnatural ingredients. Anything that doesn't come from the earth or that has chemically enhanced ingredients isn't good for your ability to naturally cleanse or feel healthy and strong.

Kicking bad habits is just as important in a healthy lifestyle as is adapting to the right ones. Just as you want to focus on eating right, exercising, and getting plenty of rest, you also want to be sure to get rid of the bad habits that are holding you back. If you can learn to manage your caffeine and alcohol intake, get rid of processed foods, and kick the smoking habit for good, your body will cleanse and feel the best it has in years!

Detox Program Do's

- Eat whole, natural foods.
- Eat only foods that will spoil, but eat them before they do.
- Eat naturally-raised meat including fish, seafood, poultry, beef, lamb, game, organ meats and eggs.
- Eat whole, naturally-produced milk products from pasture-fed cows, preferably raw and/or fermented, such as whole yogurt, cultured butter, whole cheeses and fresh and sour cream.
- Use only traditional fats and oils including butter and other animal fats, extra virgin olive oil, expeller expressed sesame and flax oil and the tropical oils—coconut and palm.
- Eat fresh fruits and vegetables, preferably organic, in salads and soups, or lightly steamed.
- Use whole grains and nuts that have been prepared by soaking, sprouting or sour leavening to neutralize phytic acid and other anti-nutrients.
- Include enzyme-enhanced lacto-fermented vegetables, fruits, beverages and condiments in your diet on a regular basis.
- Prepare homemade meat stocks from the bones of chicken, beef, lamb or fish and use liberally in soups and sauces.
- Use herb teas and coffee substitutes in moderation.
- Use filtered water for cooking and drinking.
- Use unrefined Celtic sea salt and a variety of herbs and spices for food interest and appetite stimulation.
- Make your own salad dressing using raw vinegar, extra virgin olive oil and expeller expressed flax oil.
- Use natural sweeteners in moderation, such as raw honey, maple syrup, dehydrated cane sugar juice and stevia powder.
- Use only unpasteurized wine or beer in strict moderation with meals.
- Cook only in stainless steel, cast iron, glass or good quality enamel.
- Use only natural supplements.
- Get plenty of sleep, exercise and natural light.
- Think positive thoughts and minimize stress.
- Practice forgiveness.

Detox Program Don'ts

- Don't eat commercially processed foods such as cookies, cakes, crackers, TV dinners, soft drinks, packaged sauce mixes, etc.
- Avoid all refined sweeteners such as sugar, dextrose, glucose and high fructose corn syrup.
- Avoid white flour, white flour products and white rice.
- Avoid all hydrogenated or partially hydrogenated fats and oils.
- Avoid all vegetable oils made from soy, safflower, sunflower, corn, canola or cottonseed.
- Do not use polyunsaturated oils for cooking, sautéing or baking.
- Avoid fried foods.
- Do not practice veganism; animal products provide vital nutrients not found in plant foods.
- Avoid products containing protein powders.
- Avoid pasteurized milk; do not consume low fat milk, skim milk, powdered milk or imitation milk products.
- Avoid battery-produced eggs and factory-farmed meats.
- Avoid highly processed luncheon meats and sausage containing MSG and other additives.
- Avoid rancid and improperly prepared seeds, nuts and grains found in granolas, quick rise breads and extruded breakfast cereals, as they block mineral absorption and cause intestinal distress.
- Avoid canned, sprayed, waxed, bioengineered or irradiated fruits and vegetables.
- Avoid artificial food additives, especially MSG, hydrolyzed vegetable protein and aspartame, which are neurotoxins. Most soups, sauce and broth mixes and commercial condiments contain MSG, even if not so labeled.
- Avoid caffeine-containing beverages such as coffee, tea and soft drinks. Avoid chocolate (except dark chocolate).
- Avoid aluminum-containing foods such as commercial salt, baking powder and antacids. Do not use aluminum cookware or aluminum-containing deodorants.
- Do not drink fluoridated water.
- Avoid synthetic vitamins and foods containing them.
- Do not drink distilled liquors.
- Do not use a microwave oven

3 days Sample plan

The three days of menus are approximately 1,500 calories per day. If you require more or fewer calories, you can simply alter the portion sizes, but do not skip any of the meals or snacks. You'll need to eat frequently to keep your stamina going.

Also, it's important to follow these guidelines:

- Keep an eye on absolutely everything that goes into your mouth. YES, I even want you to avoid chewing gum and breath mints.

- Drinking water is a true necessity, especially when you are cleansing. Almost all of your liquids should be pure, unadulterated water. We usually recommend about 64 ounces per day.

- Decaf green tea and hot water with lemon may be added for those people missing their warm morning mug.

- If all of these guidelines seem too daunting to take on at once, feel free to mix and match. In other words, you could follow the menus but allow yourself one small cup of coffee. Make it work for you, but remember that the more you adhere to the plan, the bigger difference you'll feel and the more effective your whole body cleanse

Day 1

Breakfast: 1 cup of steel-cut or Irish oats (measured after cooking), topped with 2 tablespoons chopped walnuts and 1 cup of fresh or frozen berries.

Snack: ½ cup plain nonfat yogurt mixed with ½ of a banana, sliced, and 2 tablespoons Grape-Nuts or other high-fiber cereal.

Lunch: Washed baby spinach leaves (or other dark green salad greens) topped with 4 ounces of grilled chicken, 8-10 sliced red grapes, sliced red onion and 2 tablespoons slivered almonds. Dress salad with fresh lemon juice and 2 teaspoons olive oil. Serve with ½ of a 6-inch whole-wheat pita pocket.

Snack: Sliced green apple with 1 ounce of cheddar cheese.

Dinner: Bake a 5-ounce piece of cod or tilapia (or other white flaky fish). Place fish in a baking dish, top with 2 teaspoons olive oil, fresh lemon juice and a pinch of sea salt and pepper. Bake at 375 for 10-12 minutes, or until cooked through; serve with ½ cup brown rice and steamed broccoli.

Day 2

Breakfast: In a nonstick skillet coated with cooking spray, make a 3-egg-white omelet filled with 2 tablespoons grated parmesan cheese and ½ cup of sliced tomatoes and onions (or other vegetable of choice). Serve omelet with a navel orange or half a grapefruit.

Snack: 1 slice of whole-grain bread topped with 1 tablespoon all-natural peanut butter or almond butter.

Lunch: 5-ounce salmon fillet grilled or poached (can purchase canned salmon if easier) served over a bed of baby arugula (or other dark green lettuce) and topped with ½ cup of chickpeas (or garbanzo beans), fresh lemon juice and 1 teaspoon olive oil.

Snack: ½ cup 1% cottage cheese (calcium-fortified if available) topped with ½ cup of fresh or frozen berries.

Dinner: Broil a lean 4-ounce ground sirloin burger (or lean ground turkey burger) and serve it on a whole-wheat English muffin topped with sautéed mushrooms and onions. Serve burger with a large mixed green salad dressed with balsamic vinegar and 1 teaspoon olive oil.

Day 3

Breakfast: Combine 1 cup of plain nonfat yogurt (look for Greek yogurt if available), 2 tablespoons flax seeds, 1 cup of fresh or frozen berries and 2 tablespoons Grape-Nuts or other high-fiber breakfast cereal.

Snack: 1 hard-boiled egg and a handful of baby carrots.

Lunch: Top a 6-inch whole-wheat tortilla with ¼ of a sliced avocado, 2 slices of tomato, 2 slices of part-skim mozzarella cheese, 1 teaspoon Dijon mustard and 1 romaine lettuce leaf. Wrap up and enjoy with a bag of fresh green or purple grapes (about 15-20 grapes).

Snack: 1 cup of skim or soy milk and 1 ounce of raw almonds (about 20 almonds).

Dinner: Bake a 5-ounce boneless skinless chicken breast with fresh lemon juice, 2 teaspoons of olive oil and 1 tablespoon of capers or sliced green olives (in oven-proof baking dish at 375 degrees for about 20 minutes -- or until cooked through). Serve chicken with a corn salad comprised of 1 cup of frozen, thawed corn niblets, 1 diced plum tomato, ¼ cup black beans, topped with a pinch of sea salt and pepper.

Tips to minimize withdrawal symptoms

Get yourself psyched to cleanse, but also be prepared. This may not be easy, but it is definitely worth it! It is really only the first one to two days that you are likely to feel any of these negative side effects, and I can assure you that by day four, you will feel better than you have in a long time!

To help combat side effects such as headaches and fatigue, try the following:

- Drink adequate water — about 64 ounces per day. This will help to ease any negative side effects.

- Add an extra piece of fruit or a very small glass of fruit juice if you are feeling extremely lethargic.

- Get at least seven to eight hours of sleep per day. If this is not possible at night, try to fit in a few catnaps during the day.

3-days radiance plan

1-day cleanse for radiance

Whether you use this body detox as a regular radiance boost or because you've just had a weekend of rich food and too much alcohol, you'll find it's really worth the effort—just take a look in the mirror 24 hours later to see the difference.

- **On waking** A large glass of hot water with a thick slice of organic unwaxed lemon

- **Breakfast** A large glass of hot water with a thick slice of organic unwaxed lemon; a large glass of Radiant Juice; a mug of nettle tea

- **Midmorning** A large glass of hot water with a thick slice of organic unwaxed lemon

- **Lunch** A large glass of Tomato Juice with Garlic and Green Onions; a mug of mint tea

- **Midafternoon** A large glass of hot water with a thick slice of organic unwaxed lemon

- **Supper** Mango, Kiwi, and Pineapple Juice; a mug of nettle tea

- **Evening** Carrot and Beet Juice

- **Bedtime** A mug of lime-blossom tea

2-day cleanse for raidiance

- Start by following the 24-Hour Cleanse for Radiance regime.

On Day 2 have:

- **On waking** A large glass of hot water with a thick slice of organic unwaxed lemon

- **Breakfast** A large glass of hot water with a thick slice of organic unwaxed lemon; a large glass of Radiant Juice; a mug of nettle tea

- **Midmorning** A large glass of hot water with a thick slice of organic unwaxed lemon

- **Lunch** A glass of Radiant Lemonade; a mug of mint tea

- **Midafternoon** A large glass of hot water with a thick slice of organic unwaxed lemon

- **Supper** A large bowl of fresh fruit salad, to include apple, pear, grapes, mango, and some berries—but not banana; a handful of raisins—chew them very slowly—and a handful of fresh, unsalted cashews; a mug of mint tea

- **Evening** A large glass of hot water with a thick slice of organic unwaxed lemon

- **Bedtime** A mug of any reputable brand of chamomile tea with a teaspoon of organic honey

3-day cleanse for radiance

When you wake up on day 4 after this cleansing regime, your body will feel lighter, your system cleaner, and your eyes and skin will have a sparkle and luster you haven't seen in ages. You'll also be overflowing with all the protective antioxidants you need and you'll almost certainly have lost more than 2 pounds in weight.

- Start by following the 48-Hour Cleanse for Radiance regime. On Day 3 have:

- **On waking** A large glass of hot water with a thick slice of organic unwaxed lemon

- **Breakfast** A large glass of hot water with a thick slice of organic unwaxed lemon; fresh fruit salad—a mixture of any of the following: apple, pear, grapes, mango, and pineapple and any berries, with 2/3 cup plain yogurt with live bacteria and a tablespoon of unsweetened muesli; a cup of weak Indian tea or herb tea midmorning 6 dried apricots; a glass of fruit or vegetable juice

- **Lunch** Watercress Soup with a chunk of crusty wholewheat bread, no butter; a cup of weak Indian tea or herb tea

- **Midafternoon** An apple and a pear

- **Supper** Zucchini Pasta; a salad of tomato, onion, and yellow bell pepper; a cup of weak Indian tea or herb tea

Recipes

Radiant Juice

- 1 large eating apple, quartered

  1 orange, peeled but with some pith

  2 large carrots, topped, tailed, and peeled if not organic

  1-inch piece of fresh gingerroot, peeled and sliced

Put all ingredients into a blender or food processor and whiz until smooth.

Tomato Juice with Garlic and Green Onions

- 8 large tomatoes

  2 fat bulbs green onions, trimmed

  4 large sprigs basil

  6 large springs oregano

Roughly chop the tomatoes and green onions and put into a blender or food processor with the leaves from the basil and oregano. Whiz until smooth.

Mango, Kiwi, and Pineapple Juice

- 1 large ripe mango, pitted

  4 kiwifruit, peeled

  1 medium pineapple, top removed

Simply put all the ingredients in a blender or food processor and whiz until smooth.

Carrot and Beet Juice

- 4 carrots, topped and tailed

  4 medium beets

  3 large sprigs basil

Put the ingredients into a blender or food processor and whiz until smooth.

Radiant Lemonade

Vitamin A is essential for healthy, radiant skin and you'll get it in abundance from the carrots in this juice. The bonus comes from the radishes—their natural constituents stimulate the cleansing function of the liver, making this the perfect juice when you've been a bit overindulgent or your digestive system seems slightly sluggish.

- 1 large carrot, topped, tailed, and peeled if not organic

  10 radishes, topped and tailed

  1 apple, quartered

  1 beet, topped and tailed

  juice and finely grated zest of 2 lemons

  up to 1-1/4 cups naturally sparkling mineral water (optional)

Juice the first 4 ingredients. Add the lemon juice and zest. If you want a longer, fizzy drink, add the mineral water.

Watercress Soup

Watercress is one of the truly great radiant foods. It's hugely antioxidant, especially protective against lung cancer, and rich in iron, which makes it a key to inner beauty.

- 1 tbsp. olive oil

  1 medium onion, finely chopped

  2 cloves garlic, finely chopped

3 bunches watercress, with stems

1 quart vegetable stock

3/4 cup plus tbsp. plain yogurt with live bacteria

Heat the oil in a large saucepan and sauté the onion gently until soft. Add the garlic and continue to cook for 2 minutes. Add the watercress and continue to cook gently until it wilts. Add the stock and simmer for about 10 minutes. Transfer to a blender or food processor and whiz until smooth. Serve hot or cold with a swirl of yogurt in each bowl.

Zucchini Pasta

- 14 oz. thin pasta, such a spaghettini

  4 medium zucchini, grated

  1-1/4-inch piece fresh gingerroot, grated

  4 tsp. extra-virgin olive oil

  4 tsp. freshly grated Parmesan cheese

  4 green onions, finely chopped

  1-1/2 cups bean sprouts

Cook the pasta in a saucepan of boiling water according to the package directions. Transfer to a large serving bowl and mix in all the other ingredients. Serve immediately.

Caffeine, sugar and white flour Eliminatation Plan

Caffeine, sugar and white flour are substances that interfere with your metabolism and brain health — and the ones people usually have the most trouble giving up and getting out of their systems.

I recommend eliminating these items from your diet in a systematic way with a detox. This may help you avoid potential withdrawal symptoms, make you feel better, and jumpstart the process to better brain function and overall health. Follow the steps below to help make the transition as simple and painless as possible.

ELIMINATE CAFFEINE PLAN

If you have been drinking caffeine for a long time, you have to get off it over a few days. Minimize your pain and the difficulty of giving up your addiction by following these detoxification steps.

Step 1: Start on a Weekend

You may want to start on a Sunday. This will allow you to take naps as needed, since your body will be recovering from the caffeine and you are liable to be fatigued.

Step 2: Reduce Your Caffeine Intake

For the first three days (Sunday, Monday and Tuesday), cut your daily intake of coffee, cola, black tea or other caffeinated beverages in half. That means if you usually have four cups of coffee in the morning, you would have two cups of coffee in the morning on Sunday, one cup on Monday and half a cup on Tuesday. Doing this helps you wean your body off the caffeine, which should reduce withdrawal symptoms.

Step 3: Drink Green Tea

For the next four days (the remainder of the week), you can drink one cup of caffeinated green tea steeped for five minutes in boiling water. You may continue drinking green tea for all its wonderful health and weight benefits. (Note that I recommend green tea as part of your morning ritual.)

You can switch to decaffeinated green tea if you want to eliminate caffeine completely. Otherwise, it is fine to have one cup of caffeinated, organic green tea every morning. The caffeine is minimal, and the health benefits are great.

Step 4: Take Vitamin C

Throughout this process, I recommend taking 1,000–2,000 mg of buffered pure ascorbic acid (vitamin C) powder or capsules. This may help you detoxify and balance your system.

Step 5: Drink Plenty of Clean Water

You should also drink at least six to eight glasses of filtered water a day. You should do this regardless of whether or not you are getting off caffeine, but it is especially important for this process because it will keep your body well hydrated and can reduce headaches and constipation, and flush toxins out of your system.

How to eliminate sugar and white flour

Eliminating sugar is hard because it's an addiction. But the physical cravings dissipate quickly once you stop eating it. Here are some tips for how you can successfully do this with a whole body cleanse.

- I recommend starting the same day you cut your caffeine intake in half.
- The tried and true method from my experience with thousands of patients: Go cold turkey from all white flour and sugar products. (Don't cheat — it will only make it worse!)
- Include protein for breakfast, such as eggs, nuts, seeds, nut butters or a protein shake.
- Combine "good" protein, "good" fat and "good" carbs at each meal. (Good fats are fish, extra virgin olive oil, olives, nuts, seeds and avocados. Good carbs are beans, vegetables, whole grains and fruit. Good proteins are fish, organic eggs, small amounts of lean poultry, nuts, soy, whole grains and legumes.)
- Don't go low-fat. Consume olive oil, olives, nuts, seeds and avocados every day. Despite commonly held beliefs, these good fats are NOT fattening.
- Eat every three hours. Snack on nuts and seeds such as almonds, walnuts or pumpkin seeds (raw or dry-roasted only). One serving is a handful or ten to twelve nuts.
- Drink at least six to eight glasses of filtered water a day.

How to ease withdrawal symptoms

The unfortunate reality is that making these changes in your diet is liable to cause a few withdrawal symptoms. They include:

- Bad breath
- Constipation
- Achy, flu-like feeling
- Fatigue
- Headaches
- Hunger
- Irritability
- Itchy skin
- Nausea
- Offensive body odor
- Sleep difficulties (too much or too little)

These symptoms are actually a good sign. They mean your body and mind are eliminating stored toxins and are finding their way to balance.

Those who consume the most caffeine, alcohol and sugar, and those who have the most food allergies, will have the most difficulty with the detoxification initially. In any event, symptoms of withdrawal usually disappear after three or four days.

What to do if withdrawal symptoms become uncomfortable

1. Make sure you drink at least six to eight glasses of filtered water daily.
2. To prevent headaches, make sure your bowels are clean.
3. If you are tired, allow more time for sleep.
4. Make sure you exercise daily to help fight off fatigue.
5. If you are hungry, have some protein in the afternoon such as a handful of nuts or seeds such as almonds, pecans, walnuts or pumpkin seeds, cooked beans, or a piece of steamed or baked fish.
6. If you're irritable or have trouble sleeping, take a combination of calcium citrate (500 mg) and magnesium citrate (250 mg) before bed.

7 days sample plan

Getting Started

This regimen is not intended to be all things to all people. Nor is it a test of will and endurance. It is designed to be a safe, useful, empowering, health guide. You can change it as necessary to meet your own needs. However, this process does require planning and preparation, so read through it and make preparations ahead of time. In addition to physical approaches, this plan equally emphasizes mind-body approaches. These can help you relax and unravel negative and unconscious mental patterns that often result in pain and discomfort.

The most important part of going through a detox program is to first ask why you are doing it. Being clear about your intentions helps avoid disappointment and expectations that are too high. Write down your reasons for going through a detox program using language that is meaningful to you.

The five basic ingredients of this detox regimen are self-reflection, exercise, sauna, nutrition, and manual-therapy. The program offered here is designed to support and enhance your own ability to heal and experience well-being. It is intended for most people, and you can do it on your own. However, first check with your primary care clinician to make certain this is a healthy option for you. We encourage you to use organic, sustainable, local, responsible, gentle, natural, whole, balanced, and easeful products and methods. These honor the global and spiritual aspect of health.

Precautions and Expectations

Healing crises commonly occur during a detoxification regimen. Common and temporary symptoms of detoxification include feeling lousy, headache, lightheadedness, diarrhea, cramps, bloating, body aches, fatigue, mood changes, and weakness. These symptoms are due to a combination of factors including the how toxins in the body are affected, low blood sugar, low fluids, electrolyte imbalance, withdrawal from various substances (such as alcohol, caffeine, sugar, nicotine), and even changes in your daily routine.

If you develop any of these symptoms, usually the best approach is to continue with the detox. However, you may need to stop or alter the detox if you experience ongoing distressing symptoms.

Dehydration is common during a detox. Make sure that you drink a lot of fluids. Address your particular needs as you go along, such as more frequent snacks, larger meals, increasing protein and healthy fats, working less, resting more, and less striving for goals. In general, continued use of prescribed daily medications is recommended. Use other medications sparingly (for example pain medication taken as needed for headaches or other problems).

Communicate with your health care provider, therapist, or other healing practitioners for any concerns that arise during the detox as needed.

In the end, you will likely find that you feel better, have more energy, and may require less

7 Day Detox

Days 1 and 2:

Eliminate meat, eggs, dairy, wheat, alcohol, caffeine, chocolate, and sugar. Eat only organic vegan foods in any arrangement, preparation, and amount using cooking oils (extra virgin olive, canola, sesame, and coconut oils) and seasonings.

Day 3:

In addition, eliminate grains, nuts, beans, and legumes. Eat only fruits and vegetables in any combination, amount, and preparation using oils and spices as needed.

Day 4:

Avoid eating any solid food. Drink plenty of water, broth, juice and tea.

Day 5: (Same as Day 3)

Days 6 and 7: (same as Days 1 and 2)

Entire Detox Week

For the entire detox week, eliminate flesh foods/meat (e.g. fish, beef, pork, lamb, poultry, etc.), refined sugars (white/brown sugar and especially high-fructose corn syrup), and artificial sweeteners such as saccharine, aspartame, and Splenda (limited use of natural sweeteners such as honey, maple syrup, and molasses are okay to use in small amounts). Also avoid alcohol, tobacco, caffeine, cigarettes, chocolate, and recreational drugs for the entire week. It is advised to avoid dairy, wheat, and eggs during the detox week as well (instead try soy/almond/rice milk, soy cheese, soy yogurt, stanol/sterol spreads). The recipes you use will guide your cooking methods, e.g. simmering vegetables into soups, steaming, sautéing, etc.

Days 1 and 2

Recommended foods for Days 1 and 2 include fresh/frozen/dried vegetables, fruit, and mushrooms (maitake, shiitake, oyster, and/or enoki, etc). Healthy grains are also recommended for days 1 and 2 (brown/wild rice, quinoa, buckwheat, oatmeal, millet, seeds, nuts, legumes, and flax seed).

Other recommendations include:

- Use cold pressed organic extra-virgin olive oil as guided by your recipes and meals.
- Add spices and healthy seasonings as guided by your recipes
- Drink 8-10 glasses of filtered water, including vitalizing-beverage, detox-broth, smoothies, and diluted juices
- Drink tea throughout the day, such as peppermint, decaf green, chamomile, licorice, ginger, rooibos, and digestive tea
- For snacks eat mixed nuts, dried and fresh fruit, vegetables and detox-broth
- Consider using herbs and supplements.
- Consider 15-30 minutes of sauna or steam room therapy
- Consider 30-60 minutes of light exercise such as walking, running, biking, skiing, jumping rope, stretching, yoga, pilates, etc
- Practice any variety of self-reflection, including meditation and breathing.

Day 3

On Day 3 also eliminate grains, nuts, seeds, legumes, beans, and mushrooms. Eat only fruits and vegetables. You can include fresh, frozen, or dried vegetables and fruit. You can eat as much of thee as you want, prepared in any healthy way. Just like Days 1 and 2, recommendations include: Olive oil

Spices and seasonings , Filtered water, tea, vitalizing-beverage, detox-broth, smoothies, and diluted juice , Optional herbs and supplements at recommended dosages, Sauna or steam room heat therapy, Light exercise, Journaling, self-reflection, or meditation.

A new suggestion to add on Day 3 is massage therapy. This can help eliminate the toxins in your body. It can also assist the body's lymphatic system, which helps balance the fluids in the body.

Day 4 (FASTING)

Eliminate all solid food (i.e., drink only water, tea, juices, and broth with modifications as needed). Most importantly, PAY ATTENTION TO THE NEEDS OF YOUR BODY! Sensitive, ill, weak, and thin people should avoid or modify this day of fasting if needed For example; you can drink more juice and broth as needed.

Other suggestions include:

- Enjoy rest and relaxation; avoid exercise and sauna use today
- Do minimal or no work today and avoid being overly active
- Stop all supplements just for today. (There's one exception. If you do the bowel cleansing described below, use the three products listed).
- Drink plenty of fluids (tea with honey, vitalizing beverage, diluted fruit/vegetable juice, and detox-broth) to replace those lost through toileting.
- Practice journaling, self-reflection, or meditation

Optional bowel cleansing regimen:

- Take 500-1000 mg of Bentonite Clay or Activated Charcoal capsules by mouth three times per day with water, only for this day of fasting (It binds toxins in the gut.)
- Drink 300 mL of Magnesium Citrate (one bottle) in the morning for bowel elimination
- Use 1-2 saline Fleet Enemas in the afternoon or evening for bowel elimination

Day 5 (Same as Day 3 except for Energy-Work)

For day 5, add back fruit and vegetables. You can eat them in any amount or combination. Prepare them using healthy recipes. Again, recommended foods include fresh, frozen, or dried vegetables and fruit (but no mushrooms, grains, seeds, beans, legumes, or nuts). Just like days 1-3, other recommendations include:

- Olive oil
- Spices and seasonings
- Filtered water, tea, vitalizing-beverage, detox-broth, smoothies, and diluted juice
- Restart the optional herbs and supplements at recommended dosages
- Sauna or steam room heat therapy
- Light exercise
- Journaling, and self-reflection, or meditation

Days 6 and 7 (Same as Days 1 & 2)

In addition to fruits and vegetables, add back mushrooms, beans, legumes, seeds, nuts, and healthy grains. You are encouraged to continue the following:

- Olive oil
- Spices and seasonings
- Filtered water, tea, vitalizing-beverage, detox-broth, smoothies , and diluted juice
- Optional herbs and supplements at recommended dosages
- Sauna or steam room heat therapy
- Light exercise
- Journaling, self-reflection, or meditation

During Your Detox-Troubleshooting Guide

Fatigue

During the first few days, this is normal and should pass by day 5-6. Try adding 1 scoop SP Whey Pro to shakes. Check medication side effects and be sure to sleep 7-8 hours. If you have tried all the above, and are still experience fatigue try removing nightshades and citrus fruits.

Cravings

If you are craving bread, pasta, soda, candy etc.

- o   This is normal at the start, but should pass by days 5-6.
- o   Consider adding Gymenma* Tablets 1 3/x per day
- o   Are you eating frequently enough? Try snacking on veggies or sipping a shake.
- o   Try adding ¼-1/2 tsp. of cinnamon to your shakes
- o   Help maintain blood sugar levels with Cataplex B or G
- o   Add starch – as cravings may be due to insufficient fats, protein

Constipation

Track your water consumption. Drinking half your body weight in ounces is the daily MINIMUM.

Additional suggestions include:

- •   Check Essential Fatty Acids (Tuna Omega 3-Oil, Linum B-6, Calamari Omega-3 Oil)
- •   Eat 1 beet per day
- •   Stop Gastro-Fiber switch to Whole Food Fiber if not already doing so
- •   Add Colax 1 3x/day before bed with full glass of water
- •   Fen-Cho – 3 3x/day with full glass of water.
- •   AF Betafood – 3 3x/day for liver congestion.
- •   Okra Pepsin – 2 3x/day between meals with water.

Headaches

Headaches can occur during the first few days of the detox program. Consider these support suggestions:

- Chew 2 Thymex Tablets
- Confirm water consumption is adequate
- AF Betafood Tablets 3 3/x day
- Cramplex Tablets 1 every hour until the pain goes away
- Confirm that you are having 1-3 bowel movements per day

Be patient as they will very likely pass in the next day or so and you should experience a new level of wellness.

Migraines

Is there nausea? This is done with Phosfood 25 drops in water hourly or more frequently as needed as soon as the first sensation of migraine comes on, or you can use Apple Cider Vinegar or fresh lemon juice 1-2Tbls. In water. Also chew 2-3 AF Betafood 3/xday

No Weight Loss

Weight loss is common on this program. If you are following the program correctly, but not experiencing weight loss, consider the following;

- If using Whey Pro Complete, you could be increasing muscle mass while losing fat.
- Check BMI vs. Body Weight
- Are you eating enough? (Review 7 day Food Diary)
- Are you "cheating" ?
- Adrenal type (apple shapes) gain weight first then lose. Be patient.
- Verify water consumption is appropriate.

Allergies - Food Intolerances

Prior to the cleanse, if you have a known whey allergy- use SP Complete Dairy Free. If you are bloated on day 4-5, you could be gaining water weight as a result of an allergy to whey. Some of the first signs that a person may be having an allergic reaction to a food include:

- A runny nose
- An itchy skin rash
- Tingling in the tongue, lips or throat
- Swelling in the throat or other parts of the body
- Abdominal pain
- Eczema
- Dizziness
- Diarrhea or vomiting
- Wheezing

*Some people notice these symptoms immediately while others don't notice them for up to

several hours after eating a particular food. Everyone is different.

Vomiting

If vomiting occurs in the first 3 days, slow down the program. Use MediHerb Liquid Ginger if feelings of nausea. If vomiting begins after adding meat to diet on day 11, think of supporting the gallbladder.

• Add 2 AF Betafood 3x/day. (Add Cholacol if patient does not have a gallbladder)

Skin Breakouts

Skin is the largest organ of the body. It is quite common for patients to note mild skin flare ups during detoxification. Patients may experience old injuries, such as wrist injuries, temporarily recur. It will usually pass quickly and is not a concern. As the body attempts to clear away stored toxins and move them out to the urine, stool and sweat, a brief inflammatory response may be encountered. This is known as "re-tracing". If the response of the body is to deal with an old injury in this fashion in order to clear it, supporting the process with Aloe Vera, Calendula Cream, on the skin can help with easing the problem.

Medications

If patient is on medication, consider possible side effects (especially with blood pressure medicines). If patient experiences dizziness upon standing- have them check with their medical doctor to possibly review their medication potency.

SAMPLE RECEPIES FOR ABOVE PLAN

Superfoods Detox Broth

Ingredients can be varied according to taste and availability.

- 1 large soup pot or kettle
- 1 strainer
- 1 large bowl or container for straining the soup
- 3-4 quarts of filtered water (Fill the pot after all ingredients are in.)
- 1 large chopped onion (white or yellow)
- 3-5 small bunches of various chopped greens (kale, parsley, cilantro, chard, or dandelion)
- 2 stalks of sliced celery
- 1 cup of fresh or dried seaweed (nori, dulse, wakame, kelp, or kombu)
- 1/2 small-medium head of chopped cabbage (any variety)
- 2 peeled carrots
- 2 stalks of peeled burdock root
- 1 large peeled daikon root
- 1 cup of squash (any variety) chopped into cubes
- 3 chopped root vegetables (especially turnips, parsnips, or rutabagas)
- 2-3 cups fresh/dried mushrooms (maitake, shiitake, oyster, or enoki)

Add all ingredients to the large pot at once and bring to a low boil for 40-60 minutes (Add water to fill.) Strain the stock to remove the solid material (Keep the liquid broth and dispose the left over solid parts.) Add salt to taste. Store in the original soup pot or a tightly sealed container to eat all week. Keep the remaining broth cooled in the refrigerator, and reheat for use. Enjoy as a sipping broth throughout the detox week, especially while fasting on Day 4.

Smoothie

Use organic ingredients when possible. This recipe makes about 1 liter, which is 4 servings (2 days worth--a glass in the AM and PM).

- About 2 tablespoons (20 mL) of organic cold pressed extra virgin olive oil
- 1⁄2 avocado
- 40g (about 3-4 tablespoons for most brands) of Whey protein powder (optional)
- 40g (about 3-4 tablespoons for most brands) of Modified Citrus Pectin (Pectasol, optional)
- 1⁄2 cup of orange juice (or 100% organic juice of choice)
- 1⁄2 cup of vanilla flavored soy milk, rice milk, or almond milk
- About 4 tablespoons (40g) of flax seed (or psyllium)
- 8-10 ice cubes (or 1⁄2 cup of filtered water)
- 1 organic banana (sliced)
- 1 organic apple or pear with peel (sliced)
- 1⁄2 cup organic frozen or fresh blueberries (and/or seasonal berries of choice)

Place ingredients in a blender and grind up until smooth, adding more water as needed. Store remaining mix in the refrigerator. Be creative, this can be varied according to taste and availability of various fruit. Enjoy 1 tall glass twice a day with or between meals

Digestive Tea

- 1⁄2 teaspoon whole fennel seeds
- 1⁄2 teaspoon whole coriander seeds
- 1⁄2 teaspoon whole cumin seeds

Add seeds to about one quart boiling water. Let the seeds steep for about ten minutes. Enjoy after meals throughout the detox week. Other recommended teas include ginger, licorice, peppermint, chamomile, rooibos, and decaf green teas.

Soup recipe, serves 4-6

Use organic ingredients when possible.

- 1 large soup pot or kettle
- 4 tablespoons of organic cold pressed extra virgin olive oil
- 1 cup barley, rinsed and strained
- 3 organic carrots, cleaned and grated or peeled
- 2 organic leeks, cleaned and sliced
- 1 bay leaf
- ½ cup fresh minced organic parsley or chervil
- 1 cup chopped mushrooms (maitake, shiitake, oyster, &/or enoki)- not the common
- Button variety!
- 1 vegetable bouillon cube
- salt to taste
- 7-8 cups filtered water

Place soup pot on medium heat and allow the pot to heat up. Pour olive oil and barley into pot and stir continuously until warm (about 5-6 minutes). Add carrots, leeks, bay leaf, chervil/parsley, mushrooms, bouillon, salt, and water. Cook the soup over low-medium heat for 45-60 minutes. (Don't boil the soup, let it simmer). Add more water if necessary. Serve hot and when barley is tender. Allow remaining soup to cool and store in the refrigerator in covered soup pot.

Detox water recipes

The water detox diet is one of the simplest detox diets around. Just by simply only drinking water throughout the day you can detox your body more efficiently than ever before. Teamed with drinking the right water and timing your drinks right there is no limit to your ability to detox the right way.

Does water detox your body?

When it comes to dieting what always seems thrown up in the air is the question, *Can water detox your body?* The question is not whether it can but how much water to drink per day to **detox your body**. You've probably been told before, but this amount is only 1.5 liters a day.

The Water Detox is one of the simplest ways to cleanse your body just by**only drinking water** you can get the detox you need to flush unwanted toxins out of your body helping you lose weight cleaner with the detox benefits of other **water diets to lose weight**.

Apple Cinnamon Detox Water

Ingredients

- A large pitcher
- Fuji apples
- Cinnamon sticks (powdered works too, I used about one teaspoon)
- Ice
- Water

This recipe has a 1:1:1 ratio, meaning you'll need 1 fuji apple and 1 cinnamon stick for 1 pitcher of water. With that said, you can leave the same apple and cinnamon stick in the pitcher for up to three days while refilling the water.

Slice a fuji apple and toss the slices into the pitcher with the cinnamon stick. Cover with ice, then fill the pitcher with water and allow it to set in the fridge for 15 minutes before drinking. Enjoy it throughout the day in the place of any juice or soda you would normally have!

Cucumber Lemon Mint Detox Water

Cucumbers are one of the most hydrating vegetables because they're mostly made up of water. Many detox programs include cucumbers on them for this very reason, and adding them to your water pulls out their minerals so you're getting an added benefit. Mix in the lemon juice and you're getting the cleansing effect of citric acid and helping to clear out the digestive system. The mint makes things taste fresh and crisp, and goes nicely with the lemon and cucumber while providing additional nutrients and benefits.

Ingredients

- 12 cups of water (3 quarts)
- 2 to 3 lemons, thinly sliced (you can also substitute limes or mix it up...use a lemon/lime combination–using organic lemons or limes is best)
- 1 small cucumber or 1/2 of a medium to large cucumber, preferably organic, thinly sliced
- 10 to 15 mint leaves. preferably organic

Rinse lemons and cucumbers very well before slicing; slice thinly. Add lemons, cucumber, and mint to pitcher. Cover with water and refrigerate at least 4 hours or overnight (the flavor will be stronger if you refrigerate overnight, but I like the lighter flavor, too). Pour in a large glass over some ice...it's very refreshing! This water tastes best the day or day after you make it.

Strawberry Detox Water

Strawberries are a great way to add a familiar and preferred flavor to most anything, and in this case it can make your water taste better while also providing antioxidants and added vitamins and minerals to your body. This particular recipe includes watermelon and rosemary as well. This makes it a great detox recipe to use in the summer when it's easier to build up a sweat, and it's only natural to have the taste of strawberries and watermelon. It will help to make your detoxing efforts more enjoyable and seem like less of a chore.

Ingredients

- 1 cup strawberries
- 2 cups watermelon, cubed
- 2 sprigs fresh rosemary
- dash of course salt
- filtered water

Directions

1. Muddle the strawberries and rosemary in a bowl.

2. Add the muddled ingredients and the watermelon to a large pitcher. Pour water over the ingredients and stir.

3. Refrigerate for 4-6 hours, and enjoy!

Apple Cider Vinegar Detox Water

Apple cider vinegar is a handy detoxing aid and it's good to keep a bottle of it in the cupboard. You can instantly improve the quality of a glass of water by adding a bit of ACV to it, but in this case they're showing you how to make a detoxifying drink from it. They're also including lemons, cucumbers, and mint, a popular combination you've seen elsewhere on our list, but the use of apple cider vinegar gives it additional properties and benefits that you won't want to miss, and that will only amplify the detoxing process.

Ingredients

- 1 lemon, thinly sliced
- 1/2 cucumber, thinly sliced
- 4 sprigs mint
- 2 quarts filtered water
- 2-6 T. apple cider vinegar (optional)

Preparation

1. Slice lemon and cucumber as thinly as possible. Divide into 2 separate quart sized bottles or mason jars.
2. Pluck mint leaves from stems and divide into jars.
3. Fill to the top with water, leaving room for as much apple cider vinegar as you want. I put 3 tablespoons into 32 oz of water, but love the taste of vinegar, so I suggest starting at 1 tablespoon and going up from there, tasting as you go and stopping when you feel like it is about to get too vinegary.
4. Refrigerate overnight.
5. Carry with you throughout the day. Enjoy!

Lemon and Cayenne Pepper Detox (Master Cleanse)

The most important part of the Master Cleanse is where you stop eating regular foods and rely only on a concoction made of organic lemon juice, maple syrup, and cayenne pepper. This is supposed to spur the body into detox mode, with the lack of food helping to give the digestive system a break and make sure that you're entirely cleared out. We've gone into detail about what you need to do in order to complete the Master Cleanse, so if you do decide on it be sure to check our guide for the best chance of success.

Ingredients

- Pure Filtered Water
- Grade B Organic Maple Syrup, Formaldehyde free
- Organic Cayenne Pepper
- Organic Lemons
- Sea salt - Unrefined, (Not iodized) or Epsom Salt

Mix all well and serve chilled

Weight Loss Detox Water (Fat Flush Water)

This is a great detox water for weight loss, and is specifically geared at getting certain fruits into your body that you otherwise might not eat. They're using grapefruit here, one of the quintessential weight loss foods that seems to always get brought up when asked which foods help to lose the most weight. Grapefruit also is a fantastic detoxing food, which is often overlooked. They use tangerines for more citrus and sweetness, and cucumbers for added minerals.

Ingredients

- 1/2 gallon water
- 6 wedges grapefruit
- 1 tangerine, sliced
- ½ cucumber, sliced
- 2 peppermint or mint leaves
- Ice

Directions

Rinse grapefruit, tangerine, cucumber and mint leaves. Slice cucumber, grapefruit, and tangerine (or peel). Combine all ingredients in a half gallon pitcher. Allow the ingredients to sit for 2 hours for maximum benefits. Drink throughout the day.

Stir & Enjoy!

SOUPS

Fat Flushing Soup

Ingredients

- 1 medium sweet potato, peeled and cut into 1" cubes (optional, 1 medium zucchini sliced into 1" round pieces)
- 3 carrots, peeled and sliced
- 1 stalk celery, diced
- 1 small yellow onion, diced
- 1 clove garlic, minced
- Kosher or sea salt to taste
- 1/2 teaspoon black pepper
- 1/8 teaspoon allspice
- 1 teaspoon paprika
- 1 bay leaf
- 2 (15 ounce) cans black beans, rinsed and drained
- 2 cups vegetable broth, low-sodium
- 1 (14.5 oz.) can diced tomatoes (no salt added)
- 4 cups baby spinach, loosely packed

Directions

Add all ingredients, except spinach, to the slow cooker. Cover and cook on low 6 to 8 hours, or until the vegetables are tender. Add spinach, stir and continue cooking just until wilted, approximately 5 minutes. Serve and enjoy!

Tip: If you prefer a thicker stew, after 5 hours of cooking, simply remove 1 cup of soup, along with ingredients, mash ingredients with a fork, return to the slow cooker, stir and continue cooking 1 to 3 hours. Stovetop Method: Follow the same instructions above for prep, cover, and simmer until veggies are tender, approximately 2 hour. Stir every 15 minutes to prevent sticking. Add spinach at the end of cooking time, remove from heat, cover and allow spinach to wilt before serving.

VEGETARIAN HOT AND SOUR SOUP

Ingredients

- 1 oz. dried mixed mushrooms
- 8 cups water
- 3 tablespoons sherry cooking wine
- 1/4 cup apple cider vinegar
- 2 tablespoons soy sauce
- 1-1/2 teaspoons kosher salt
- 1 tablespoon grated ginger
- 1 pound extra firm tofu, cut into 1/2 inch cubes
- 2 tablespoons cornstarch
- 2 eggs, lightly beaten
- 6 scallions, trimmed and thinly sliced
- 1/4 teaspoon white pepper
- Pure sesame oil, for serving

Place the dried mushrooms in a bowl and cover with 2 cups of boiling water. Cover and allow to sit for at least 1/2 hour. While mushrooms reconstitute, prepare the other ingredients.

Remove the mushrooms from the hot water and reserve the liquid for the soup. Slice the mushrooms thinly.

In a soup pot, combine the remaining 6 cups of water with the reserved liquid from the mushrooms and the sliced mushrooms. Bring to a gentle boil over medium-high heat. Add the sherry, vinegar, soy sauce, salt, ginger and tofu. Reduce the heat and allow to simmer uncovered for about 10 minutes. In a small bowl, whisk the cornstarch with about 3/4 cup of hot broth from the soup pot until cornstarch is dissolved. Pour the mixture back into the soup pot, stirring to distribute. The soup should thicken slightly. While stirring constantly, drizzle the beaten eggs into the hot soup. Add the scallions and white pepper and cook for another minute or two. Serve hot with a drizzle of sesame oil on top.

Spicy green soup

Ingredients (serves 2):

- 4 celery stalks
- 1 yellow onion
- 1 green bell pepper
- 5 big handfuls of spinach
- 2 garlic cloves
- 1/2 teaspoon cardamom
- 1/2 teaspoon ground ginger
- 1/2 teaspoon ground cumin
- 1 teaspoon dried mint
- 1 l water
- cream or coconut milk (optional)
- sea salt and freshly ground black pepper

Directions:

Boil water in a pot and add sea salt to your taste. You will need 1-1.5 l water - you can boil 1.5 l, cook your veggies and before blending the soup pour out excess liquid not to have your puree too thin.

Chop your celery, onion, bell pepper and spinach and add them to the pot. Cook the vegetables over medium heat covered with a lid for 15 minutes until they soften.Turn off the heat, add 2 whole garlic cloves and blend your soup - raw garlic will give it a nice contrasting hot note.Pour the soup into the plates, add some cream or coconut milk if you want, sprinkle with some more freshly ground black pepper and enjoy!

Radish Leek Soup Recipe

Ingredients

- 3/4 lb radishes, halved
- 3 yukon potatoes, peeled and cubed
- 2 leeks
- 32 oz chicken broth
- 1-2 tsp Braggs Sea Kelp Seasoning
- 2 tbs butter
- 1 cup whole milk
- Salt and pepper to taste

Directions

1. Separate the tops of the leeks. Slice up the stalk. Wash out the leaves well and set aside.

2. Add butter to pot turn up the heat then add everything but the chicken broth, leaves, and milk. Mix it up then add in the chicken broth. Stand the leaves up in the pot. Bring soup to boil and reduce to a simmer

3. Let simmer for one hour or until vegetables are tender. Discard leak tops

4. Cream the soup with a blender. Mix in the milk. Salt and pepper to taste

Lentil, Kale, and Sweet Potato Stew

- 1 can low sodium diced tomatoes
- 2 cups low sodium chicken broth (or veggie broth)
- 1 cup lentils, dried green
- 1 large sweet potato, cut into small cubes
- 1 yellow onion, diced
- 1 green or red pepper, diced
- 1 tbsp curry powder
- Pinch garam masala, cumin (optional)
- 3 cloves garlic
- 1 bunch kale, coarsely chopped
- 2 cups water (more or less, depending on if you want it soupier or stew)
- 1 small zucchini, quartered and diced (optional)

Saute onion in a small amount of olive oil (add a splash of water if things start to stick). Add sweet potato, garlic, and curry powder after 3 minutes. Saute for about 5 more minutes, until everything is tender. Add can of tomatoes, lentils, broth, and water. Simmer on low heat for 45 minutes or until lentils are tender. Add kale and red pepper at the end, so they don't get soggy, and cook for about 10 more minutes! Done!

Healthy Detox Soup

Ingredients:

- 2 medium leeks, cut in half, cleaned well, and cut into small pieces
- 4 cloves of garlic, crushed into a paste
- 1 serrano pepper, half of seeds removed, thinly sliced
- 4 carrots, scrubbed clean, skins on, cut into rough chunks
- 4 celery stalks, cut into rough chunks
- 3 small rutabagas, peeled and cut into medium dice
- 3 small zucchini, diced
- 8 cups water
- 3 roma tomatoes, with seeds and skin, diced
- 2 cups pinto beans, I used dried ones that I cooked before hand, used cooking liquids in soup
- 2 bunches of kale, thinly sliced
- 1 juice of 1/2 lemon
- maldon salt, to taste
- fresh cracked black pepper, to taste

Method

1. Heat a large pot over medium heat.
2. Add the leeks, garlic, and serranos.
3. Sweat over low heat for 5 minutes, stirring often.
4. Add carrots, celery and the rutabagas. Cook for about 3 minutes.
5. Add the water, tomatoes and pinto beans, simmer over low heat for at least 30 minutes.
6. The longer, the better the flavor is.
7. 15 minutes before serving stir in the kale and zucchini
8. Cook for 5 minutes.
9. Stir in lemon juice.
10. Season with salt and pepper to taste.
11. Serve.
12. Eat.

Kale and Lentil Soup (Vegan)

Ingredients

- 8 cups **Vegetable Broth**
- 1 ½ cups **Red Lentils** (rinsed)
- 2 **Carrots**
- 2 **Onions** (diced)
- 1 bunch **Kale** (remove stem and roughly chop)
- 1 clove **Garlic**
- ¼ teaspoon **Red Pepper Flakes** (optional)
- 1 tablespoon **Parsley** (chopped then measured)
- Zest ½ **Lemon**

Instructions

1. Add the veggie broth, lentils, carrots, onions, kale, and garlic to a large pot

2. Bring to a boil and let cook until the lentils are tender (about 15-20 minutes)

3. Stir in the red pepper flakes, parsley, and lemon zest

4. Serve and enjoy!!

GERSON'S HIPPOCRATES SOUP

<u>Ingredients</u>

- 1 big or 2 small fresh organic leeks
- 1 kg fresh organic potatoes
- 1,5 kg organic fresh tomatoes
- 800ml water
- 1 large organic onion
- 1 medium organic celery knob
- 2 garlic cloves
- 1 small parsley root
- few sprigs of organic parsley
- pinch sea salt

Don't peel any of the vegetables (apart from garlic) as many of the minerals and nutrients are stored directly beneath the skin. Scrub carefully and cook slowly at low heat for 3 hours with water, mash, garnish with parsley and eat. Let the soup cool before storing. Keep in air-tight container in the refrigerator and consume in no more than 48 hours. To reheat, simmer over stove.

BROCCOLI AND PEA POTAGE WITH THYME

Ingredients

- 1 tablespoon olive oil
- ¼ cup chopped green onions
- 1 shallot, finely chopped
- 1 lb broccoli, cut into florets
- 1 tablespoon fresh thyme leaves
- ¼ teaspoon salt
- ½ teaspoon ground black pepper
- 3 cups vegetable broth (homemade preferred)
- ¾ cup frozen peas, thawed
- ¾ cup cooked green or brown lentils
- 1-2 cups fresh spinach, cleaned, stems removed, and torn into smaller pieces

Instructions

1. Heat oil in large saucepan over medium-high heat until hot. Add green onion and shallots and cook 3-5 minutes, stirring frequently. Add broccoli, thyme, salt and pepper, and sauté 5 minutes. Add broth and bring to a boil. Add peas and lentils. Cook an additional 5-10 minutes, or until vegetables are tender. Cool slightly. Add spinach to soup pot.

2. Working in batches, puree soup in blender or food processor until smooth and creamy. Return soup to pot, and heat over low until soup is hot.

3. Taste for salt and pepper, adding more as desired. Serve hot.

Detox Green Machine Soup

Ingredients

- 1 lb green beans
- 8 celery sticks
- 4 lb zucchini
- 2 bunches spinach
- 1 yellow onion
- 5 cloves garlic
- 1 bunch basil
- 1 bunch parsley

Instructions

1. Steam green beans, celery and zucchini until very soft, about 15 minutes.
2. Add onion, spinach and garlic and cook for 5 miuntes.
3. If you desire a very thick soup, drain excess water.
4. Add parsley and basil and puree until smooth. Season with salt and pepper to taste.

Gingery Noodle Soup

Ingredients:

- 2 spring onions
- 1 knob of ginger, my piece had about the size of two walnuts
- 2 cloves of garlic
- 2 fennel bulbs
- 1 tbsp sesame oil
- 1 tbsp vegetable oil (I usually have sunflower or canola oil at home)
- 3 tbsp soy sauce
- 1 tablespoon miso
- 1 bouillon cube

Slice the spring onions, garlic and fennel into thin slices. Grate the ginger right into the pot you want to make your soup in. (I started grating the ginger with the skin still on, less waste of ginger and time. It works well, and you really don't have any hard chunks in the soup) Add the white part of the onions and the oil, turn on medium-high heat and let it all heat up. Sauté for a minute or two, then add the fennel and garlic. Sauté for another minute, add the soysauce. Add about 2 litres of water and the miso and bouillon. Bring to a boil and cook for at least 5 minutes.

In another pot bring water to a boil. Cook the noodles according to the instructions on the package. I cooked my soba without salt for about 5 minutes, drained them, rinsed them well with cold water and added them into the soup. Turn off the heat, wait another minute and serve the soup in bowls. Sprinkle some of the green parts of the spring onions onto each bowl. I also added some Nanami Togarashi (Japanese 7-ingredients red pepper powder), or just use regular red pepper flakes to make it a bit more spicy.

Eat the noodles using chopsticks and drink the soup, feels and tastes way better than with a spoon.

Detox/Beans & Greens Soup

Ingredients

- 3/4 cup dry cannellini beans
- 2 tablespoons olive oil
- 1 onion, finely diced
- 4-8 cloves garlic, minced (I like a lot)
- 1.5 teaspoons sea salt
- 1 teaspoon black pepper
- 2 bay leaves
- 1 teaspoon fresh thyme
- 3 tablespoons vegetable base
- 2 teaspoons tomato paste
- 6-7 cups water
- 4 cups collard greens, finely shredded
- fresh parsley to garnish
- grated parmesan to garnish

Instructions:

1. Cover beans with about 3 cups of cold water. Cover and let soak overnight.
2. Drain and rinse beans. Set aside. (skip steps 1&2 if using canned beans)
3. In large stockpot, heat olive oil on medium heat. Add onion, saute for 5 minutes. Add garlic, and saute until mixture starts to turn golden brown. Add salt, pepper, thyme, bay leaf, and vegetable base. Stir, cooking for one more minute.
4. Add tomato paste, water, and beans. Stir to combine and bring to a boil. Reduce heat to medium low, cover, and cook for 20 minutes.
5. Add greens, and continue to cook for 20 minutes or until beans are soft. Add water if soup becomes too thick.
6. Remove bay leaves. Garnish with chopped fresh parsley and grated parmesan. Serve with crusty bread.

NO-Chicken Soup

Makes a large pot of soup

- 1 pound dry chickpeas
- 1 cup brown rice
- 2 cubes natural vegetable bouillon
- 3 tablespoons extra virgin olive oil
- 1 pound carrots, medium dice
- ½ pound celery, medium dice
- 1 medium onion, medium dice
- kosher salt and freshly ground black pepper

2 Days Before:
Rinse the chickpeas in cold water. Soak overnight at room temperature covered in water.

Day Before:
Rinse and drain the soaked chickpeas. Add the drained chickpeas and 4 quarts of water to a large pot. Bring to a simmer over medium heat. Maintain a very low simmer covered for one hour. Add the brown rice and bouillon to the chickpeas and simmer for an additional hour. Allow to cool and store in an airtight container overnight in the refrigerator.

To finish the soup:
Heat a large pot over medium heat. Add the olive oil, carrots, celery, and onion to the pot. Season with salt and pepper. Saute until the vegetables are tender and are just beginning to brown, about 15 minutes. Add yesterday's chickpea-rice-broth mixture to the pot and some additional water if the soup looks too thick. Bring to a boil and simmer for five minutes. Season with additional salt if necessary. Serve and enjoy!

Roasted Butternut Squash and Apple Soup

Yields 8 dinner-sized portions

- 2-3 pound butternut squash, cubed in 1-inch pieces
- 4 large sweet apples (such as Gala or Honeycrisp), cubed in 1-inch pieces
- 8 ounces mushrooms, cut in half
- 1 cup (about 4 stalks) celery, cut into 2-inch pieces
- 1 large onion, cut into fourths
- 1/4 cup olive oil
- 4 cups low-sodium chicken or vegetable broth
- 1 cup apple juice
- 2 teaspoons salt + extra to taste
- 1 teaspoon black pepper + extra to taste
- 1/2 teaspoon nutmeg
- 1 teaspoon cinnamon
- 1/2 teaspoon red pepper flakes, optional (for a little extra kick)
- Pumpkin seeds, optional (for garnish)

Preheat oven to 425 degrees F (220 degrees C).

In a large bowl, mix together the butternut squash and onion with 1/8 cup of olive oil. Stir to coat evenly. Place the vegetables in a large baking pan and bake for 30-40 minutes, or until squash is fork tender.

Meanwhile, mix together the apples and mushrooms with the remaining olive oil. Place on another baking pan and bake for 15-20 minutes, or until soft and fragrant.

In a large soup pot, place roasted vegetables and add chicken broth and apple juice. Using a an immersion blender, puree vegetables (alternatively, you may use a blender and puree vegetables with the liquid. This may take 2-3 batches). If the soup is too thick, additional chicken broth or water can be added to thin it out to your desired consistency. Simmer the soup over medium-low heat and season with spices, adding more or less to suit your taste.

Serve warm and garnish with pumpkin seeds, parsley or thyme, and a splash of cream.

Detox Green Soup Recipe With Broccoli

Ingredients:

- 1 tablespoon olive oil
- 2 cloves of garlic, chopped
- 2 tablespoons diced onion
- 1 inch of fresh ginger, peeled and chopped
- 4 cups fresh broccoli, cut up
- 1/2 pound of fresh spinach leaves
- 3 parsnips, peeled, cored, chopped
- 2 ribs of celery, trimmed, chopped
- A handful of fresh parsley, roughly chopped
- Fresh water, as needed
- Sea salt and ground pepper, to taste
- Lemon or lime juice

Instructions:

Using a large soup pot, heat the olive oil over medium heat and stir in the garlic, onion, and ginger to season the oil. Add the broccoli, spinach, parsnips, celery and parsley, and stir a bit until the spinach wilts and collapses. Add just enough water to cover the vegetables. Remember the spinach will cook down quite a bit, so don't add too much water at first. You can always thin the soup later, if you need to.

Bring to a high simmer, cover the pot, and reduce the heat to a medium simmer. Cook for fifteen minutes or so until the veggies are softened.

Use an immersion blender to puree the soup.

Taste test. Does it need brightening? Add a squeeze of citrus.

DETOX SOUP: CLEANSING MISO, BEET, ASPARAGUS

ingredients

- 1 tablespoon olive oil
- 1/3 cup onion of choice diced
- 1/3 cup chopped celery
- 1 cup peeled, chopped beet
- 1/2 cup chopped carrot
- 1 cup chopped asparagus (bases removed, tips left whole)
- Some fresh scallions, chopped
- Large handful flat-leaf fresh parsley, chopped
- 1 tablespoon minced ginger
- 5 cups water
- Salt (about 1 teaspoon) to taste
- 3 tablespoons miso paste of choice
- A little minced jalepeño or chile pepper (to taste)

DIRECTIONS:

1. Heat the oil in a large pot over medium-high heat. Add the onion and sauté for a few minutes until begins to brown. Add the celery and scallions and half the parsley and sauté for another minute.

2. Add the water, beet, carrot, ginger, salt and pepper of choice. Increase the heat to high. Bring to a boil, reduce the heat to medium/low, cover and simmer for 10 to 15 minutes.

3. While that cooks, remove a ladle of the hot water from the pot and place in a small bowl on the side. Add miso paste to the small bowl and stir/mash in until fully combined (refer to image in post). Now add the dissolved miso to the soup pot. You can't skip this step and just add the miso directly to the main pot of soup – it will clump and never fully incorporate.

4. Add the asparagus and cook for another 5 minutes. Remove from the heat when asparagus are bright green and still firm. Stir in remaining parsley. Place in bowls and serve warm.

Roasted Pumpkin Soup

Ingredients:

- 820gm pumpkin, diced into half-moon pieces
- 1 onion, peeled and dice
- 8 cloves of garlic, peeled and smashed
- 450ml water
- 200ml fresh milk
- 1 sprig of fresh Rosemary
- 2 tbsp olive oil
- salt and pepper to taste

Steps:

1. Preheat the oven at 150 deg C. Diced the pumpkin into half-moon shape pieces. Remove the seeds. Sprinkle a tablespoon of olive oil over the pumpkin. Roast it for 15 minutes with a sprig of fresh Rosemary.

2. When time's up, leave the pumpkin to cool. Remove the skin and cut it into cubes.

3. Heat a tablespoon of olive oil in a sauce pan. Saute onion and garlic for 2 minutes. Add the pumpkin and saute for another 3 minutes. Pour in 350ml of water and bring to a boil. Close the lid and leave it simmering for 8 minutes. By this time the pumpkin should be turn soft. Off the fire, and leave the soup to cool down a bit.

4. Pour the soup into blender and blend till smooth. Reheat the soup with 100ml of water and 200ml of milk. Add salt and pepper to taste. Serve hot.

Sweet Pea, Ginger and Mint Soup

- 1 bag frozen sweet peas (16 oz)
- 1 medium shallot, diced
- 2 T fresh ginger, minced
- 1/4 c fresh mint
- 1 T olive oil
- Water
- salt & pepper

In a medium sauce pan heat the olive oil on a low/med setting. Add shallots and ginger and sautee for about 3 minutes.

Next add 3/4 of the bag of frozen peas, stirring for 1 minute.

Add enough water to cover the peas and cook over medium heat for 10 minutes.

Let the soup cool enough to place in a blender. Add soup and fresh mint and puree the combination. Add salt and pepper to taste.

Return the soup to the pan and add the last of the peas. They will defrost in the warm soup but will retain a bit of pop.

Carrot, Cumin and Ginger Detox Soup

Serves 4

- 1 medium onion, sliced
- 2.5cms/1inch knob of ginger peeled and chopped
- 1 tablespoon oil
- 1 kg/2 pound bag carrots, peeled if desired, cut into rough chunks
- 1 teaspoon cumin powder
- 1 litre/1 quart vegetable or chicken stock
- 1 tablespoon cumin seeds to sprinkle

Step 1 - Sautee onion and ginger in oil until translucent and then add carrots and cook for about 5 minutes. Add stock, cumin powder and simmer for about 45 minutes to an hour until carrot is very soft (if you don't want to cook it for that long, cut the carrot up into smaller pieces). Check for seasoning and add salt and pepper to taste.

Step 2 - Puree soup in a blender and serve with a teaspoon of cumin seeds sprinkled on top.

SUPER SMOOTHIES

Tropical Green Energy

This smoothie recipe is loaded with tropical fruits and rich in antioxidants and Vitamin C. The Matcha Green Tea powder adds a subtle taste and is one of the richest sources of the antioxidant EGCG, which Helps metabolism and speed up weight loss. If you are looking for a tropical treat high in vitamin C and powerful antioxidants – blend up a tropical green energy.

- ½ Cup Orange Juice (Not From Concentrate)
- ½ Cup Coconut Milk (No Sugar Added)
- 2 tbsp Matcha Green Tea Powder
- ½ Frozen Banana
- ½ Cup Frozen Mango

Directions:
1. Add all ingredients into a blender and whiz
2. Enjoy!

Popeye's Weight Loss Punch

Make sure you are buying the no sugar added almond milk as your liquid base, as this boasts just 40 calories per Cup! Much lower than regular milk and better for your health. Mixed Berries and Spinach leaves provide you with tons of fiber and nutrients that will energize you, keep you full, and keep your body running like a machine. Chia seeds provide a great source of Omegas and are high in dietary fiber to keep you full. This is one incredibly well rounded smoothie that gives you all of the nutrients you need. Great for lunch or Dinner when you are trying to lose weight and get healthy!

- 1 Cup Almond Milk
- 1 Cup Mixed Berries (Strawberry, Blackberry, Blueberry)
- ½ Cup Spinach Leaves
- 1 Scoop Whey Protein
- 1 tbsp Chia Seeds

Directions:

1. Add all ingredients into a blender and whiz

2. Enjoy

Tropical Weight Loss Recovery

When you are working out to lose weight you need to make sure that you are feeding your body the proper "recovery formula." This smoothie is high vitamins with oranges, pineapple, and banana.Whey Protein and L-Glutamine will combine to give your body a great boost of amino acids and protein and help to keep you full without the addition of carbohydrates. This smoothie has under 400 calories and is absolutely delicious after an intense cardio session or summer day.

- 1 Cup Orange Juice
- ½ Cup Pinneapple
- ½ Frozen Banana
- 1 Scoop Whey Protein

Directions:

1. Add all ingredients into a blender and whiz

2. Enjoy!

Fruit Protein Meal Replacement

This is a fantastic recipe that includes vitamin C, Potassium, iron, calcium, amino acids and lean protein! Makes for an incredible meal replacement shake for weight loss that packs a huge health punch! Greek yogurt is high in fiber and low in fat and sugar making it an ideal choice for those seeking weight loss and nutrition. This fruit protein meal replacement smoothie blends together for a delicious and smooth combination.

- 1 Cup Orange Juice
- ¼ Cup Fat Free Greek Yogurt
- ½ Frozen Banana
- ¼ Cup Raspberry
- 1 Scoop Whey Protein

Directions:

1. Add all ingredients into a blender and whiz

2. Enjoy!

Breakfast in a Blender

No more pancakes and bacon. Throw this recipe in the blender and you will reap some amazing weight loss and health benefits. This smoothie will keep you full until lunch time and packs a great combination of vitamins and nutrients with slow digesting carbohydrates. Slow digesting carbohydrates and fiber are key for weight loss because they will keep you full for long periods of time. This is the perfect breakfast choice for someone seeking optimal health and weight loss.

- 2/3 Cup Coconut Milk
- 2/3 Cup Almond
- ¼ Cup Greek Yogurt
- ½ Cup Oatmeal or Rolled Oats
- ¼ Cup Strawberry
- ½ Frozen Banana

Directions:
1. Add all ingredients into a blender and whiz
2. Enjoy!

Pina Colada Health Twist

Now you can enjoy this tropical treat without all of the guilt of a real pina colada. This makes for a great meal replacement shake in the summer time or for anyone who enjoys pina coladas. This tropical smoothie has all the bold tropical flavors you want in a smoothie with coconut, banana, and pineapple. Coconut Oil has been well known for its health properties and energy inducing properties. Whey protein gives you a nice protein add in that will keep you full and energized. Coconut Milk is low in calories and high in health! Blend and enjoy this tropical treat.

- 1 Cup Coconut Milk
- 1 Tbsp Coconut Oil
- ½ Frozen Banana
- ¼ Cup Frozen diced Pineapple
- 1 Scoop Whey Protein

Directions:
1. Add all ingredients into a blender and whiz
2. Enjoy!

Antioxidant Powerhouse

This smoothie is absolutely loaded with antioxidants and cancer fighting polyphenols! Pomegranate, Blueberry, and red grapes are absolutely loaded with antioxidant and disease fighting properties.If you are looking for a big health boost while you enter flu season or before you go on vacation, make sure to blend up an antioxidant powerhouse.

- 1 Cup Pomegranate Juice (Not From Concentrate)
- ¼ Cup Blueberry
- ¼ Cup Red Grapes
- ¼ Cup Blackberry
- 2 tbsp Chia Seeds

Directions:
1. Add all ingredients into a blender and whiz
2. Enjoy!

Tropical Green Tea Power

The tropical green tea power will give you a great big boost of energy and nutrition. Combining the powerful antioxidant properties of matcha green tea with the omega rich flax seeds – this smoothis has everything you need for optimal health and energy. Throw in banana and mango and you have a smoothie that is also rich in vitamins and fiber. Tropical green tea power is sure to deliver great results.

- 1 Cup Almond Milk (No Sugar Added)
- 1 Tbsp. Matcha Green Tea Powder
- ½ Frozen Banana
- ½ Cup Frozen Mango Chunks
- 1 tbsp Ground Flax Seed

Directions:
1. Add all ingredients into a blender and whiz
2. Enjoy!

Chocolate Peanut Butter Weight Loss

For all of us who are on a diet and craving the combination of peanut butter and chocolate – finally a delicious and healthy alternative! Believe it or not this smoothie has under 400 calories! Peanut butter and low fat chocolate whey protein make this a delicious combination that will keep you full for long periods of time. L-Glutamine is a great recovery aid for keeping your health and energy levels high when you are training to lose weight.

- 1 Cup Almond Milk
- 2 Tbsp Peanut Butter
- ½ Frozen Banana
- 1 Scoop Whey Protein (Chocolate)

Directions:
1. Add all ingredients into a blender and whiz
2. Enjoy!

The Greek God

This is a very simple and delicious smoothie recipe. Almond Milk is a great low calorie liquid base. Greek yogurt will add in a big punch of protein and fiber. Raspberry and Strawberry will provide a nice antioxidant boost with all of the vitamins and fiber you need for optimal health.

- 1 Cup Almond Milk
- ½ Cup Greek Yogurt
- ½ Cup Raspberry
- ½ Cup Strawberry

Directions:
1. Add all ingredients into a blender and whiz
2. Enjoy!

Digestive Helper

Keeping you regular is an important component to optimal health and weight loss. Prune juice is rich in vitamins and dietary fiber. Greek Yogurt adds additional fiber, calcium and protein. Blackberry and blueberry are vital for your health and are two of the top antioxidant fruit's in the world.

- 1 Cup Prune Juice
- ¼ Cup Greek Yogurt
- ¼ Cup Blueberry
- ¼ Cup Blackberry

Directions:
1. Add all ingredients into a blender and whiz
2. Enjoy!

Cherry Berry Energy Thriller

This is one tart and fruity smoothie that has a wide range of antioxidant and vitamin properties. A true berry lover will enjoy this smoothie. Mixed Berries and Cherry's make a delicious and tart combination. Blueberry Juice is rich in antioxidants and will provide a big burst of energy. Chia seeds are rich in omega's and provide great all around nutrition.

- 1 Cup Blueberry Juice (Not From Concentrate)
- ½ Cup Frozen Cherry's
- ½ Cup Frozen Mixed Berries (Raspberry, Strawberry, Blackberry)
- 1 tbsp Chia Seeds

Directions:
1. Add all ingredients into a blender and whiz
2. Enjoy!

Morning Smoothie Tart

This tart and delicious smoothie will pep you right up in no time! The delicious tastes of orange juice, strawberry, banana and lime makes this a healthy start to any day. Limes are actually very healthy and help to "alkalize" the body, which is key for optimal health. Chia seeds give you some dietary fiber to keep you full until lunch time. This smoothie is delicious and less than 300 calories. A perfect start to any day.

- 1 Cup Orange Juice (Never from Concentrate)
- ½ Cup Frozen Strawberry
- ½ Frozen Banana
- Juice from ½ a lime
- 2 Tbsp. Chia Seeds

Directions:
1. Add all ingredients into a blender and whiz
2. Enjoy!

Apples and Antioxidants

An apple a day keeps the weight gain away! Apples are high in all of the essential vitamins and nutrients and will keep you full because they are high in fiber. Coconut milk is a great liquid base, and the orange juice will give you a big burst of Vitamin C. Matcha green tea is known to be one of the top antioxidant and metabolism boosters due to its high EGCG profile.

- ½ Cup Orange Juice
- ½ Cup Coconut Milk
- ½ Apple
- ¼ Cup Frozen Pineapple
- 1 Tbsp. Matcha Green Tea Powder

Directions:

1. Add all ingredients into a blender and whiz

2. Enjoy!

Tropical Nutrition Phenomenon

This is one of my favorite smoothie recipes because it packs in a ton of Vitamin A and K along with tropical and delicious fruits. Kale and spinach are two of the most nutrient dense foods in the world, and the somewhat bitter taste of this is covered up perfectly by the pineapple and mango. This is one delicious and nutrient dense tropical treat.

- 1 Cup Coconut Milk
- ¼ Cup Spinach
- ¼ Cup Kale
- ¼ Cup Frozen Pineapple
- ¼ Cup Frozen Mango

Directions:
1. Add all ingredients into a blender and whiz
2. Enjoy!

Coconut ICED Green Tea

This is one of my favorite green tea recipes of all time. Matcha Green tea is one of the healthiest forms of green tea, and helps with weight loss because of its metabolism boosting properties. is a great choice for a natural sweetener. Enjoy this iced green tea guilt free without any added sugar or fat!

- 1 Cup Coconut Milk
- 2 Tbsp Matcha Green Tea
- 2 Tbsp Natural Sweetener
- 5-6 Ice Cubes

Directions:
1. Add all ingredients into a blender and whiz
2. Enjoy!

Kiwi Colada

Coconut Oil is a great source of energy and antioxidants. Ground Flax seed in the recipe blends great and is a vital source of important Omega 3's. Cranberry is rich in vitamins and antioxidants and blends deliciously with pineapple. Enjoy this unique and tangy smoothie and cheers to your health!

- 1 Cup Coconut Milk
- ½ Kiwi
- 2 Tbsp. Coconut Oil
- ½ Cup Frozen Pineapple
- 1 tbsp Ground Flax Seed

Directions:
1. Add all ingredients into a blender and whiz
2. Enjoy!

Banana's Gone Wild

This is a rich and delicious smoothie that will keep you full and provide tons of vitamins and minerals. Banana's gone wild has a rich and tropical taste and has an almost ice cream like consistency with its frozen banana, almond milk, and frozen mango. An incredibly healthy smoothie recipe that also packs in fiber and omegas with chia seeds as well as healthy fats with coconut oil.

- 1 Cup Almond Milk
- 1 Frozen Banana
- 1 Tbsp Coconut Oil
- ¼ Cup Frozen Mango
- 2 Tbsp Chia Seeds

Directions:

1. Add all ingredients into a blender and whiz

2. Enjoy!

Staying Lean with Greens

This smoothie recipe is rich in vitamins and antioxidants and will help to alkalize your body with the addition of kale, spinach and avocado. Apples are high in fiber and vitamins and make this a delicious and nutritious add in to this powerhouse health recipe. This is one of the healthiest and most "healing" recipes on the list, and is a great choice for weight loss, overall health, and energy.

- 1 Cup Almond Milk
- ¼ Cup Kale
- ¼ Cup Spinach
- ½ Avocado
- 1 Apple
- 2 Tbsp. Sweetener

Directions:
1. Add all ingredients into a blender and whiz
2. Enjoy!

Green Grapple

The green grapple has a unique and fruity taste. Green tea has been known as a great metabolism boosting drink helping tons of consumers lose weight. It makes the perfect liquid base for a weight loss drink. Red grapes give this a sweet taste with a great concentration of polyphenols. Red apples are another vital source of vitamins and fiber.

- 1 Cup Green Tea
- ½ Cup Red Grapes
- ½ Red Apple
- 2 tbsp. Sweetener
- 5-6 Ice Cubes

Directions:

1. Add all ingredients into a blender and whiz

2. Enjoy!

Revenge of the Tropical Antioxidants

This recipe is sure to please! Green tea is a known metabolism booster and watermelon goes perfect with the subtle taste of green tea. Red grapes and mango give this smoothie additional fiber and vitamins. Ground flax seed is a must for optimal health because of its high level of omegas. This recipe is perfect for weight loss, and metabolism.

- 1 Cup Green Tea (Home Made Non Sweetened)
- ½ Cup Watermelon Chunks
- ¼ Cup Red Grapes
- ¼ Cup Frozen Mango
- 2 tbsp. Ground Flax Seed

Directions:

1. Add all ingredients into a blender and whiz

2. Enjoy!

Tropical Carrot Antioxidant

Carrot Juice is extremely rich in vitamin A and is a perfect choice for many smoothie bases. This smoothie is extremely rich in vitamins A and C making it a perfect health boosting snack at any time of the day. Blend smooth and enjoy the wonderful health boost.

- 1 Cup Carrot Juice (Never From Concentrate)
- ¼ Cup Frozen Mango
- ½ Frozen Banana
- ¼ Cup Frozen Pineapple

Directions:

1. Add all ingredients into a blender and whiz

2. Enjoy!

The Green Beet

This is another extreme health booster. Beets have wonderful health boosting properties and are one of my favorite vegetables. Green tea gives this drink a big metabolism boost and is a light and subtle calorie free liquid base. Strawberry and Raspberry conceal the taste of the beet and provide necessary vitamins and nutrients.

- 1 Cup Green Tea
- ½ Beet Root
- ¼ Cup Raspberry
- ¼ Cup Strawberry
- 2 tbsp. Sweetener

Directions:

1. Add all ingredients into a blender and whiz

2. Enjoy

Cucumber Lime Refresher

An extremely easy and delicious drink to enjoy on a hot day. This drink will stimulate weight loss through its green tea base, and optimal health with alkalizing cucumber and lime. One of my favorite smoothies to enjoy on a hot summer day.

- 1 Cup Green Tea
- ½ Cucumber
- 1 Squeezed Lime
- 4-5 Ice Cubes

Directions:

1. Add all ingredients into a blender and whiz

2. Enjoy!

Strawberry Lemonade Nutrition

Now you can enjoy lemonade without all of the added sugar and calories. Green tea gives it a metabolism boosting base. Fresh squeezed lemon juice gives this smoothie a tart and tangy lemonade flavor. Vitamin rich strawberry is the perfect complement to the tart lemon flavor. is a healthy all natural sweetener that will perfect this recipe and give it a sweet after taste.

- 1 Cup Green Tea
- 1 Fresh Squeezed Lemon
- ½ Cup Frozen Strawberry
- 2 tbsp.

Directions:

1. Add all ingredients into a blender and whiz

2. Enjoy!

Vitamin Carrot Punch

An intriguing vitamin A-C rich combination of carrot, apple and orange, the vitamin carrot punch provides optimal health with a fruity twist. Ground flax seeds cap off this amazing recipe with the perfect amount of omega fatty acids and fiber.

- 1 Cup Carrot Juice
- ½ Apple
- ½ Orange
- 2 tbsp. Sweetener
- 2 Tbsp. Ground Flax Seeds

Directions:

1. Add all ingredients into a blender and whiz

2. Enjoy!

Health Booster

Could this be the perfect combination of weight loss and antioxidants? Combining three of the richest antioxidant sources in the world with metabolism boosting green tea, the health booster is a smoothie you can enjoy at any time of the day. I have this smoothie 2-3 days a week and my body thanks me each and every time!

- 1 Cup Pomegranate Juice
- ¼ Cup Strawberries
- ¼ Cup Wild Blueberry
- 1 Tbsp Matcha Green Tea

Directions:

1. Add all ingredients into a blender and whiz

2. Enjoy!

Health Freak

The health freak is a delicious blend of nutrition. Blending deliciously with coconut milk is creamy avocado, apples, and baby carrots. This smoothie recipe will help you alkalize and detox your body while providing optimal energy levels. Loaded with vitamin K from the carrots and Vitamin C from the apple - the Health Freak is the perfect blend of vitamins and minerals to help your body run like a machine.

- 1 Cup Almond Milk
- ½ Avocado
- 1 Apple
- 5 Baby Carrots
- Ice Cubes

Directions:

1. Core the apple and prepare ½ an avocado

2. Add all ingredients into a blender and whiz

3. Enjoy!

Kiwi-Tastic

This is a fruity and fiber filled recipe that provides a huge amount of vitamins, minerals and antioxidants. Blackberry and Cherry combine to give this a tart and tangy flavor while Kiwis are rich and fiber filled. Coconut milk is a healthy and low calorie base that brings this recipe together for a healthy formula.

- 1 Cup Coconut Milk
- ½ Kiwi
- ¼ Cup Cherry
- ¼ Cup Blackberry
- 2 Tbsp Sweetener

Directions:

1. Add all ingredients into a blender and whiz

2. Enjoy!

Berry Breakfast

Don't let its pink-liciousness fool you. The berries turn on detoxifying enzymes and ginger stimulates digestion in this recipe.

- 1 cup frozen unsweetened raspberries
- 3/4 cup chilled unsweetened almond or rice milk
- 1/4 cup frozen pitted unsweetened cherries or raspberries
- 1 1/2 Tbsp honey
- 2 tsp finely grated fresh ginger
- 1 tsp ground flaxseed
- 1-2 tsp fresh lemon juice

Directions:

1. Add all ingredients into a blender and whiz

2. Enjoy!

The Super Green

Powerful detox action masquerades as another delicious shake from *Prevention*'s Lori Powell (it's pictured here with the Berry Breakfast Smoothie.) The celery and parsley that contribute to its bright green color are diuretics that help rinse toxins from your system. Kale and mango are superfoods bursting with nutrition that support your cleanse.

- 1¼ cups chopped kale leaves (stems and tough rib removed), preferably Lacinato (also known as dinosaur)
- 1¼ cups frozen cubed mango
- 2 medium ribs celery, chopped
- 1 cup chilled fresh tangerine or orange juice
- ¼ cup chopped flat-leaf parsley
- ¼ cup chopped fresh mint

Directions:
1. Add all ingredients into a blender and whiz
2. Enjoy!

Hale to the Kale

These powerful detox smoothies keep in the fridge for a day, so feel free to make several rounds at once,

- ½ pear
- ¼ avocado
- ½ cucumber
- ½ lemon
- handful of cilantro
- 1 cup kale (packed)
- ½ inch ginger
- ½ cup coconut water
- 1 scoop protein powder (hemp, pumpkin or pea works great!)
- pure water

Directions:
1. Add all ingredients into a blender and whiz
2. Enjoy!

Sweet Spirit

Don't fear its dark color and mossy smell: spirulina—a form of micro-algae—is a mega-healing detox agent.

- ½ banana
- ½ cup blueberries
- ¼ avocado
- ½ cup almond milk
- 1 tsp spirulina
- 1 scoop vanilla protein powder (hemp, pumpkin or pea works great!)
- Pure water

Directions:
- 1. Add all ingredients into a blender and whiz
- 2. Enjoy!

Alkalinity Bliss

A single teaspoon of chia seeds packs almost 2 grams of fiber!

Serves 1-2

- ½ pear
- ¼ avocado
- 1 packed cup spinach
- ¼ cup coconut water
- 1 cup almond milk
- 1 tsp chia seeds
- 1 scoop protein powder (hemp, pumpkin or pea works great!)
- pure water

Directions:

1. Add all ingredients into a blender and whiz

2. Enjoy!

Belly Soother

Treat your tummy to a healthy dose of probiotics, found in tangy kefir.

Serves 1-2

- 1 cup papaya
- 1 cup coconut kefir, coconut yogurt or cultured coconut milk
- juice from ½ lime
- 1 tbsp raw honey

Directions:
1. Add all ingredients into a blender and whiz
2. Enjoy!

Smooth Operator

This greenie features the crunchy root vegetable jicama, which is rife with vitamin C.

Serves 1-2

- 5 large Romaine lettuce leaves
- ½ Granny Smith apple
- ¼ avocado
- ½ cucumber
- ½ cup jicama
- handful of cilantro
- 1 whole lime
- 4 scoops of hemp protein
- 1 medjool date
- pure water

Directions:

1. Add all ingredients into a blender and whiz

2. Enjoy!

Morning Glorious

- 1 large cucumber
- A fistful of kale
- A fistful of romaine
- 2 or 3 stalks celery
- 1 big broccoli stem
- 1 green apple, quartered
- ½ peeled lemon, quartered

Directions:

- 1. Add all ingredients into a juicer
- 2. Enjoy!

Crazy Sexy Goddess

"The avocado, cucumber, greens, and coconut water will shower your cells in alkalinizing goodness," Carr says. "An alkaline inner environment helps your body's systems operate optimally."

- 1 avocado
- 1 banana
- 1 cup blueberries
- 1 cucumber
- A fistful of kale or romaine or spinach
- Coconut water (or purified water)
- Stevia, to taste, and/or a sprinkle of cinnamon or some cacao (optional)

Directions:

- 1. Add all ingredients into a blender and whiz
- 2. Enjoy!

Strawberry Fields

Berries of shortcake fame are also great for a detox. "Strawberries are phytonutrient factories, supplying your body with a bounty of anti-inflammatory and antioxidant nutrients,"

Serves 2

- 3 cups cashew or nondairy milk of your choice
- 2 cups fresh strawberries
- 1 tablespoon lemon zest
- 1 small orange, peeled
- 1 banana
- 1½ cups loosely packed spinach

Directions:
1. Add all ingredients into a blender and whiz
2. Enjoy!

The Sicilian

This hearty, spicy drink fills you up when your tummy is grumbling. "Celery's fabulous phytochemical, phthalide, makes this veggie a heart helper. "Phthalide relaxes the smooth muscles of the arteries, which helps to lower blood pressure."

- 6 carrots
- 3 large tomatoes
- 2 red bell peppers
- 4 cloves garlic
- 4 stalks celery
- 1 cup watercress
- 1 cup loosely packed spinach
- 1 red jalapeño, seeded (optional)

WASH and prep all ingredients.
JUICE all ingredients.

Lemon-Blueberry

Aimee Follette, Executive Chef and owner of gluten-free, vegan, and raw restaurant <u>Sun In Bloom</u>, serves up the next three smoothies. This super-simple recipe boosts immunity.

Serves 1

- 1 cup alkaline water
- ¼ cup organic blueberries
- 1 organic lemon (whole).

Directions:
1. Add all ingredients into a blender and whiz
2. Enjoy!

Strawberry Goji Lassi

"This is one of my absolute favorite Sun In Bloom recipes

- 1 cup of coconut kefir water
- 1 frozen banana
- ¼ cup frozen strawberries
- 3 Tbsp Goji berries

Directions:

- 1. Add all ingredients into a blender and whiz
- 2. Enjoy!

Blueberry Ginger

This gluten-free smoothie is packed with antioxidants.

Serves 1

- 1 cup almond milk (or milk of choice)
- ¼ cup blueberries
- 1 frozen banana
- 3 Tbsp ginger juice

Directions:

- 1. Add all ingredients into a blender and whiz
- 2. Enjoy!

Mint Apple Berry

Guzzle this in the morning, and the protein will keep you full until lunch.

Serves 1-2

- ½ green apple
- 2 tablespoons of Manitoba Harvest Hemp Hearts
- 8 fresh mint leaves
- 3-4 leaves of organic green leaf lettuce
- ¼ cup organic fresh or frozen berry blend
- 8-12 oz pure water

Directions:

- 1. Add all ingredients into a blender and whiz
- 2. Enjoy!

.

Sensual Detox

Sip yourself sexy.

Serves 1-2

- 1 tablespoon of Essential Living Foods cacao powder
- 2 tablespoons of hemp seeds
- 4-5 red endive leaves
- pinch of Essential Living Foods green stevia
- ¼ cup of organic fresh or frozen dark red cherries
- 8-12 oz pure water

Directions:

1. Add all ingredients into a blender and whiz

2. Enjoy!

Green Machine

Barley grass, a nutrient-dense grain, can help soothe inflammation and pain.

Serves 1-2

- 1 green apple
- 1 teaspoon of Essential Living Foods barley grass juice powder
- 1 lemon
- 1 cucumber, peeled
- 3-4 leaves of red leaf lettuce
- ¼ cup of organic fresh or frozen mango
- 8-12 oz pure water

Directions:

1. Add all ingredients into a blender and whiz

2. Enjoy!

Liver Cleanser

Serves 1

- 50% kale
- ¼ cup parsley
- 1 small beet (scrubbed and quartered)
- 1 apple (core and seeds removed)
- 1 lemon (peeled)
- ½" chunk of fresh ginger
- 1 Tbsp chia seeds
- Water to the max line

Directions:
1. Add all ingredients into a blender and whiz
2. Enjoy!

Glowing NutriBlast

Pumpkin seeds pack magnesium, a mineral that might improve your sleep and keep migraines at bay.

Serves 1

- 25% spinach
- ½ small cucumber
- 1 pear (core and seeds removed)
- 1 lemon (peeled)
- 1 orange (peeled)
- 1 Tbsp pumpkin seeds
- Water to the max line

Directions:

1. Add all ingredients into a blender and whiz

2. Enjoy!

Warrior Tonic

Serves 1

- 1 cup almond milk
- 1-2 Tbsp maca powder
- 1 scoop of your favorite vanilla protein powder
- 2 Tbsp chia seeds
- 1 organic ripe banana
- 1 Tbsp coconut oil
- 1 Tbsp lucuma powder (natural sweetener)
- 1-2 Tbsp cacao nibs

Directions:
1. Add all ingredients into a blender and whiz
2. Enjoy!

Clear Skin Sip

It's a gluten-free, golden ticket to a clear complexion! Coconut kefir restores radiance with live probiotics. Parsley oxygenates, cucumber revitalizes, coconut oil moisturizes, lime provides toning vitamin C, and mint packs vitamin A, which strengthens skin tissue and helps reduce oily skin.

Serves 1

- 1 cup coconut kefir
- ½ cup packed flat-leaf parsley (leaves and stems)
- 1 cucumber, seeded if you don't have a high speed blender
- 1 apple
- 1 Tbsp coconut oil
- 1 lime
- 2 Tbsp fresh mint leaves, or to taste

Directions:

1. Add all ingredients into a blender and whiz

2. Enjoy!

Berry Elixir

We're gaga for antioxidant-rich goji, since studies have shown it might reduce fatigue and stress.

Serves 1

- 1 cup coconut milk
- 1 cup blueberries
- ½ cup raspberries
- ½ cup blackberries
- 2 Tbsp Goji berries (soaked for 15 minutes) or 1 tablespoon of Goji powder
- 1 Tbsp coconut oil
- 1 Tbsp ground flaxseed
- 2 dates, pitted

Directions:
1. Add all ingredients into a blender and whiz
2. Enjoy!

Fountain of Youth

Another great alkalyzer. Plus, blue-green algae is chock full of protein and provides essential amino acids.

Serves 1

- 1 cup coconut water
- 3 stalks of kale
- handful of spinach
- ½ cup packed flat-leaf parsley (leaves and stems)
- ½ cup cilantro (leaves and stems)
- 1-2 green apples
- ¼ tsp fresh grated ginger
- 1 heaping Tbsp wild blue-green algae (jack it to 2 tablespoons if you really want some potency!)

Directions:
1. Add all ingredients into a blender and whiz
2. Enjoy!

Cranberry Cleanser

Sip this wintry detox juice to keep your kidneys strong.

Serves 1

- ½ cup cranberries
- 1 large celery stalk
- 1 cucumber
- 1 apple
- 1 pear
- Handful of spinach

JUICE all ingredients.

The "Fat Flush" Juice

If a flatter belly is on your wish list, start with this ultra-cleansing juice.

Serves 1

- 1 medium organic red beet
- 3 medium organic carrots
- 1 organic radish
- 2 organic garlic cloves
- large handful of organic parsley

JUICE all ingredients.

Detox and weight reduction salads and meals

Cran-Quinoa Salad

Serves 4

- Salad:
  1 cup uncooked quinoa
  1/4 cup dried cranberries
  2 scallions, finely chopped
  2 cups mixed greens such as spinach and arugula
- Dressing:
  1/4 cup cashews
  1/8 cup pine nuts
  2 tsp miso paste
  1/4 tsp agave nectar
  1/2 cup water
  3 Tbsp freshly squeezed lemon juice
  2 cloves garlic, minced
  1 Tbsp lemon zest
  1/4 tsp crushed red pepper
  1/4 tsp sea salt
  1/4 tsp black pepper

Cook quinoa according to package instructions. While quinoa
cooks, combine all dressing ingredients in a blender; process until smooth.
Add water if dressing is too thick. In a large serving bowl, combine cooked
quinoa, dried cranberries, scallions and mixed greens; gently toss with
caesar dressing to coat. Serve chilled.

Raspberry Salad

Serves 6

4 large red potatoes
1 cup fresh raspberries
4 cups loosely packed mixed leafy greens such as arugula or baby spinach
1/2 cup snap peas
1/2 large red onion, thinly sliced
1 Tbsp coconut oil, melted
1/2 tsp honey
1 Tbsp finely chopped fresh sage
1 Tbsp sesame seeds
1/4 tsp sea salt
1/4 tsp crushed red pepper
1/4 tsp black pepper

BOIL a large pot of lightly salted water over medium heat; add potatoes and cook for 20 minutes or until tender. Remove from heat; drain and run under cool water for 1 minute. Dice potatoes and place in a large bowl.

ADD remaining ingredients; gently toss to combine.

TRANSFER to serving bowls; serve warm.

Snow Crab Black Rice

Serves 4

2 cups cooked black rice
1 Tbsp lemon zest
1 Tbsp harissa sauce
1 Tbsp olive oil
2 scallions, thinly sliced
1/4 cup finely chopped fresh parsley
1/4 tsp sea salt
1/4 tsp pepper
8 fresh crab cocktail claws
1/4 cup Greek plain yogurt

COOK crab claws in a large pot of boiling water for 2-3 minutes or until pink and well done. Drain water; set crab claws aside.

In a large bowl, **COMBINE** all ingredients except crab cocktail claws; gently toss to combine.

TRANSFER rice mixture into four serving bowls, place two crab claws into each bowl.

SERVE warm with a tablespoon of yogurt.

Honey Quinoa

Serves 4

1 1/2 cups uncooked quinoa
1 Tbsp honey
1/3 cup fresh cilantro, finely chopped
1/3 cup honey roasted peanuts
Juice of 1 fresh orange
2 tsp fresh orange zest
2 scallions, thinly sliced
1/4 tsp sea salt
1/4 tsp freshly ground pepper

COOK quinoa according to package instructions. Remove from heat and immediately transfer to a large bowl. Add honey; gently toss to combine. Set aside covered for 10 minutes to allow honey to soak.

COMBINE remaining ingredients and add to bowl.

TRANSFER to serving bowls. Serve warm or chilled.

Lemon Squash Salad

Serves 4

1 medium yellow squash, cut into 1/2 inch pieces
2 cups cooked teff (gluten-free grain)
1 cup steamed baby spinach
2 scallions, thinly sliced
1/2 medium red onion, thinly sliced
3 Tbsp fresh lemon juice
1 tsp balsamic vinegar
1 Tbsp lemon zest
2 Tbsp extra virgin olive oil
2 tsp ground chia seeds
1 large head Bibb lettuce
1/2 tsp sea salt
1/4 tsp freshly ground black pepper
1 Tbsp finely chopped fresh cilantro, for garnish

In a large bowl, **COMBINE** squash, teff, spinach, scallions and onion.

To make the dressing, **WHISK** lemon juice, balsamic vinegar, lemon zest, olive oil, chia seeds, sea salt and pepper in a separate small bowl.

POUR dressing over squash mixture; gently toss to combine.

TEAR apart pieces of Bibb lettuce and place into serving dishes. Evenly divide teff mixture on top. Garnish with fresh cilantro, if desired.

Watermelon Salad

Serves 4

2 cups yellow watermelon, cut into 1/2 inch chunks
2 cups pink watermelon, cut into 1/2 inch chunks
1 cup fresh blueberries
6 fresh strawberries, quartered
3 cups packed fresh baby mixed greens
2 tsp fresh lemon zest
1/2 tsp sea salt
1/2 tsp freshly ground white pepper
2 Tbsp sesame seeds
1 tsp Dijon mustard
2 Tbsp apple cider vinegar
2 Tbsp Barlean's Flax Oil

In a large bowl, **COMBINE** watermelon, blueberries, strawberries, mixed greens and lemon zest; set aside in the fridge to chill for 10 minutes.

WHISK remaining ingredients in a small bowl. Allow to chill in the refrigerator for 5 minutes.

REMOVE salad and dressing from fridge. Drizzle dressing over salad; gently toss to combine. Serve chilled.

Sweet Berry Quinoa

Serves 4

1 cup uncooked quinoa
1 pint blackberries
1 pint raspberries
2 Tbsp finely chopped fresh basil
2 cups mixed greens
1 scallion, finely chopped
2 Tbsp balsamic vinegar
1 tsp stevia powder
1/2 tsp sea salt
1/2 tsp freshly ground pepper
1 Tbsp extra virgin olive oil
2 Tbsp fresh lemon zest
2 Tbsp Barlean's ground flax seeds

COOK quinoa according to package directions. Remove from heat and set aside to cool for 20 minutes.

COMBINE cooked quinoa, blackberries, raspberries, basil, mixed greens and scallions; gently toss to combine in a large bowl. Place in the refrigerator to chill for 25 minutes.

In a separate bowl, **WHISK** remaining ingredients.

REMOVE quinoa salad from the fridge; gently toss with balsamic dressing. Serve chilled with additional lemon zest.

Coconut Black Rice

Serves 4

1 1/2 cups uncooked black rice
1 pint fresh raspberries
1 lb. fresh asparagus, ends removed
1 Tbsp fresh lemon zest
2 scallions, finely chopped
2 Tbsp shredded coconut
1/2 tsp sea salt
1/4 tsp freshly ground pepper
2 Tbsp Barlean's Coconut Oil

COOK black rice according to package instructions; drain and set aside.

RINSE raspberries and set aside. Using kitchen scissors, cut asparagus into 1/2-inch pieces. In a medium sized pot, steam asparagus in a steamer basket for 8 minutes or until asparagus is tender. Remove from heat; set asparagus aside to cool for 5 minutes.

Gently **TOSS** cooked rice, asparagus, lemon zest, scallions, coconut, sea salt and pepper together in a large bowl. Place in the refrigerator for 20 minutes.

REMOVE from fridge; fold fresh raspberries into salad and gently toss to combine. Drizzle with coconut oil. Serve chilled.

Blackberry Salad

Serves 4

1 pint fresh blackberries
1 Tbsp fresh lemon zest
4 cups packed mixed greens
1 Tbsp fresh dill, finely chopped
1 scallion, chopped
Juice of 1 large lemon
2 Tbsp red wine vinegar
1 Tbsp Barlean's Flax Oil
2 Tbsp sesame seeds
1/2 tsp sea salt
1/2 tsp freshly ground black pepper

COMBINE blackberries, lemon zest, mixed greens, dill and scallions in large bowl. Set aside.

WHISK together lemon juice, vinegar, oil, sesame seeds, sea salt and pepper in a small bowl. Pour dressing over blackberry salad; gently toss to combine.

SERVE at room temperature or chilled.

Mushroom Rice Salad

Serves 8

3 Tbsp extra virgin olive oil
2 cloves garlic, finely chopped
2 cups shiitake mushroom caps, thinly sliced
2 large carrots, chopped
1 shallot, chopped
2 celery stalks, chopped
1/4 tsp sea salt
1/2 tsp freshly ground pepper
3 cups black rice, cooked according to package instructions
2 Tbsp balsamic vinegar
2 scallions, thinly sliced

PREHEAT oven to 325 degrees F.

HEAT olive oil over medium heat in a large skillet. Add garlic and stir-fry until fragrant, about 30 seconds. Add mushrooms and sauté for 1 minute.

ADD the carrots, shallot, celery, sea salt and pepper. Stir-fry until vegetables are tender, about 5-7 minutes. Add the cooked black rice and balsamic vinegar. Mix well to combine.

TRANSFER the rice mixture into a 9 x 13 inch baking dish. Cover loosely with tin foil; bake for 30 minutes or until set.

REMOVE from oven; top with scallions and serve.

Pesto Red Rice

Serves 6

1 1/2 cups uncooked red rice
2 cups broccoli florets
1 lb. asparagus, cut into 1 inch pieces
2 cloves garlic, peeled
2/3 cup pine nuts, toasted, plus more for serving
¾ tsp sea salt
½ tsp freshly ground black pepper
Juice of 1 lemon
1/4 cup extra virgin olive oil
1 cup dairy-free plain yogurt
1 yellow bell pepper, diced
3 chives, finely chopped

COOK red rice according to package directions.

As rice cooks, **STEAM** the broccoli and asparagus. Then, bring 1 cup water to a boil in a large pot. In small batches, add broccoli and asparagus to pot, cover and cook for 1 minute or until bright green and crunchy. Drain the vegetables in a colander and run under cold water. Repeat with remaining broccoli and asparagus. Set aside.

To make the pesto, **COMBINE** cooked broccoli, asparagus, garlic, pine nuts, sea salt, pepper and lemon juice in a food processor. Drizzle in olive oil and spoon in yogurt; pulse until smooth.

TOSS cooked red rice with the pesto mixture. Thin with warm water for desired consistency.

SERVE topped with additional pine nuts, diced yellow bell pepper and chives.

Red Rhubarb Quinoa

Serves 4

- For salad:
  2 heads Bibb lettuce
  1 1/2 cups red quinoa, cooked
  1 cup Daikon radish, shredded
  1 cup purple cabbage, shredded
  1/2 medium red onion, sliced
  1 large carrot, shredded
  1 large McIntosh apple, sliced
  1 pint cherry tomatoes
  1 cup organic salsa
  1/2 cup canned pumpkin
  1/3 cup salted pistachios

- For dressing:
  1/4 cup honey
  1/3 cup green tea, brewed
  4 stalks rhubarb, sliced
  1/2 shallot, sliced
  1/3 cup apple cider vinegar
  1 tsp. spicy brown mustard
  1/2 cup Barlean's flax oil

COMBINE the first eight salad ingredients in a large salad bowl.

To make the dressing, **COMBINE** agave nectar and brewed green tea in a medium saucepan and bring to a boil; add rhubarb and shallot. Boil for 4 more minutes, stirring often. Reduce to a simmer; add apple cider vinegar and cook for another 12 minutes or until liquid is reduced by half and rhubarb is tender. Remove from heat; set aside to cool.

TRANSFER rhubarb mixture to a food processor with remaining dressing ingredients; pulse until smooth. Serve atop salad; top with a spoonful of pumpkin, salsa and pistachios.

Maple Slaw Salad

Serves 4

- For salad:
  4 cups fresh baby spinach
  1/4 cup arugula
  1/2 small head Napa cabbage, shredded
  1/2 small head red cabbage, shredded
  2 large carrots, shredded
  5 large radish, shredded
  1 cup fresh basil leaves
  1/4 cup finely chopped fresh parsley
  1 tsp lemon zest
  1/4 cup pistachios
- For dressing:
  3 Tbsp olive oil
  1/3 cup shallots
  2/3 cup apple cider vinegar
  1 tsp Barlean's chia seeds
  1/4 cup pure maple syrup
  2 Tbsp freshly squeezed lemon juice

COMBINE all salad ingredients in a large salad bowl; set aside.

WHISK together dressing ingredients in a medium skillet; cook for 15 minutes. Remove from heat; drizzle atop salad and serve.

Tahini Plain Jane

Serves 4

- For salad:
  4 cups Romaine lettuce, chopped
  1 large Roma tomato, sliced
  1/2 medium red onion, thinly sliced
  2 cucumbers, sliced

- For dressing:
  1/2 cup tahini paste
  2 Tbsp balsamic vinegar
  1 clove garlic, minced
  2 Tbsp poppy seeds
  1 cup green tea, brewed
  2 Tbsp grapefruit juice
  1/6 tsp sea salt
  1/6 tsp freshly ground pepper

COMBINE all salad ingredients in a large serving bowl. Place in the refrigerator to chill until ready to serve.

COMBINE all dressing ingredients in a blender; puree until smooth. Transfer to a sealed container. Refrigerate for 2 hours before serving.

POUR dressing over salad right before serving.

Vegan Ginger Caesar

Serves 4

1 1/2 lbs. medium Brussels sprouts
4 cups mixed greens (spinach, radicchio, etc.)
1/2 cup arugula
3/4 cup rice milk
1/2 cup pumpkin puree
1 tsp white balsamic vinegar
2 tsp Barlean's ground flax seeds
1 ripe avocado, pitted and peeled
1 Tbsp maca powder
1/4 tsp fresh lemon juice
1 tsp honey
1/6 tsp curry powder
1/6 tsp fresh ginger root
1/8 tsp ground cinnamon
1/4 tsp sea salt

On the stovetop over medium heat, **STEAM** Brussels sprouts for 10 minutes or until tender and bright green. Remove from heat and transfer to a large salad bowl. Add mixed greens and arugula.

ADD remaining ingredients in a blender; pulse until smooth. Pour dressing onto salad and gently toss to combine. Serve chilled.

Mint Brussels Sprouts

Serves 2

1 lb. medium Brussels sprouts
2 Tbsp sherry vinegar
2 Tbsp Barlean's ground flax seeds
1/2 Tbsp ground chia seeds
1 tsp chlorella
1/4 tsp cumin
1/6 tsp fresh ginger
2 Tbsp Barlean's flax oil
1 small Vidalia onion, thinly sliced
1/4 tsp sea salt
1/4 tsp pepper
4 cups fresh mixed greens
2 cups fresh baby arugula
1/2 cup torn fresh mint leaves
2 Tbsp pistachios, finely chopped
1 tsp fresh lemon zest, for garnish

FILL a large bowl with ice water. Blanch Brussels sprouts for 3 minutes in a large saucepan of boiling salted water. Transfer to the ice bath. Drain and pat Brussels sprouts dry.

BEAT sherry vinegar with flax seed, chia seeds, chlorella, cumin and ginger in a large bowl. Slowly whisk in flax oil until emulsified. Add Brussels sprouts and onions; gently toss to coat, then season with sea salt and pepper.

ARRANGE mixed greens and arugula on a platter and top with the dressed Brussels sprouts, mint leaves and pistachio nuts. Gently toss to coat. Garnish with lemon zest.

Thyme Fennel Salad

Serves 4

2 bulbs of fennel with fronds, thinly sliced
1 medium red onion, sliced
1 tsp fresh marjoram, chopped
1 1/2 cups arugula
2 tsp fresh thyme, finely chopped
1/4 cup Barlean's flax oil
2 tsp freshly squeezed orange juice
2 Tbsp white balsamic vinegar
1/4 tsp sea salt
1/4 tsp freshly ground pepper
1/3 cup cashews, finely chopped
1/2 tsp fresh orange zest

COMBINE fennel, fronds, onion, marjoram and arugula in a large bowl and gently toss to combine.

In a small bowl, **COMBINE** thyme, flax oil, fresh orange juice, balsamic vinegar, sea salt and pepper; whisk well. Add cashews and gently toss to coat.

TRANSFER salad onto serving plates. Sprinkle with orange zest and serve with thyme vinaigrette on the side.

Basil Avocado Salad

Serves 2

1 large fennel bulb, slice stalks and bulbs into 1/2 inch pieces
2 cups fresh baby arugula
1 ripe avocado, peeled, pitted and sliced
1 large carrot, finely chopped
Juice from 1 organic lemon
2 Tbsp extra virgin olive oil
1/4 tsp lemon zest
4 fresh basil leaves, finely chopped
1/4 tsp sea salt
1/4 tsp freshly ground black pepper
2 Tbsp Barlean's chia seeds
1/4 cup cashews

FILL a large bowl with ice water.

BRING a large pot of salted water to a boil. Add fennel and cook for 3 minutes. Drain fennel and immediately submerge into ice bath. Set aside for 3 minutes. Drain.

TRANSFER fennel to a large serving bowl; pat dry. Add avocado and carrot.

DRIZZLE salad with lemon juice, lemon zest, oil, basil, sea salt and pepper. Gently toss to coat.

DIVIDE salad between 2 serving dishes. Top with ground chia seeds and cashews. Serve at room temperature.

Apple Pumpkin Soup

Serves 4

2 Tbsp coconut oil, melted
2 Granny Smith apples, cut into 1/4 inch pieces
1 cup brewed red zinger tea, chilled
1/4 cup freshly squeezed orange juice
1 (15 oz.) can pureed pumpkin
1/4 cup salted peanuts
1/3 cup dried cherries, finely chopped
1/4 cup finely chopped fresh mint
1/4 cup finely chopped fresh basil
1/4 tsp stevia powder
1/4 tsp freshly ground pepper
1 tsp coconut flakes
2 Tbsp orange zest, plus more for garnish

COMBINE all ingredients in a large bowl; gently toss to combine. Divide soup evenly among four serving bowls. Serve chilled or at room temperature.

GARNISH with more orange zest if desired.

Vegan Avocado Soup

Serves 4

3 ripe avocadoes, peeled, pitted and chopped
2 cups plain dairy-free plain yogurt
1/3 cup raw cashews
1/3 cup finely chopped fresh cilantro
1/3 cup Vidalia onion, chopped
1 Tbsp white balsamic vinegar
1 cup green tea, brewed and chilled
1 tsp. sea salt
1/4 tsp. freshly ground pepper
2 chives, finely chopped

COMBINE avocado, yogurt, cashews, cilantro, onion, balsamic vinegar, green tea, sea salt and pepper in a food processor and pulse until smooth.

REMOVE avocado soup from processor and transfer to a covered bowl. Place in the refrigerator to chill for 2 hours.

LADLE soup into four bowls; serve chilled. Garnish with chives.

GF Ginger Pasta Salad

Serves 4

1 lb. gluten-free pasta
1/2 cup almond milk
1/4 cup dried cranberries
1 Tbsp pine nuts, toasted
1/4 cup finely chopped fresh parsley
1 tsp ground cinnamon
1 tsp fresh ginger
1 Tbsp fresh orange zest
1/4 tsp sea salt
1/4 tsp freshly ground white pepper

COOK pasta according to package instructions. Remove from heat, drain in a colander and transfer to a large bowl.

ADD remaining ingredients to pasta; gently toss to combine.

SERVE warm.

Creamy Bean Dip

1 clove garlic, peeled and minced
2 cans (15 oz. each) white beans, drained and rinsed
1/3 cup extra virgin olive oil
2 Tbsp balsamic vinegar
1 Tbsp fresh lemon juice
1 Tbsp fresh basil, finely chopped
1/4 tsp sea salt
1/4 tsp black pepper

COMBINE garlic, white beans, olive oil, vinegar, lemon juice, basil, salt and pepper in a food processor and pulse until smooth. Transfer dip to a serving bowl.

SERVE with shrimp, crab or raw vegetables.

Almond Egg Hummus

1 (15 oz. can) chickpeas, drained and rinsed
1 large red bell pepper, diced
2 large eggs, hardboiled
1 Tbsp. tahini
1 Tbsp. fresh dill, finely chopped
2 Tbsp. fresh lemon juice
1/4 tsp. hot sauce
1/4 tsp. sea salt
1/4 tsp. black pepper
1/4 cup slivered almonds

PULSE all ingredients except almonds in a food processor until smooth.
Transfer to a serving bowl. Add almonds; mix to combine.

SERVE dip with whole grain crackers, spread on toast or inside a sandwich.

Honey Greek Yogurt

Serves 2

2 cups Greek plain yogurt
1/4 tsp vanilla extract
1 tsp ground cinnamon
2 Tbsp slivered almonds
2 Tbsp ground flax seeds

COMBINE yogurt with vanilla extract in a large bowl and mix well to combine. Divide yogurt mixture among four serving bowls and top with cinnamon, almonds and flax seeds.

SERVE chilled.

Blueberry-Coconut Baked Steel Cut Oatmeal

Ingredients

- 1 1/2 cups (260 grams) Steel Cut Irish Oats
- 1/2 teaspoon ground Ginger
- 1/2 teaspoon fine Sea Salt
- 1 teaspoon Baking Powder
- 4 cups (950 ml, 32 ounces) unsweetened Vanilla Almond Milk
- 2 cups (480 ml, 16 ounces) light unsweetened Coconut Milk
- 1 1/2 (240 grams) cups fresh Blueberries (frozen OK too, do not thaw first)
- 1/4 cup (47 grams) unsweetened dried Blueberries
- 1/4 cup (22 grams) unsweetened Coconut Flake
- Vanilla Stevia Drops or your favorite natural sweetener to taste
- 2 cups (360 grams) fresh or frozen Blueberries
- Toasted Nuts
- Coconut Flake
- Whipped Cream (vegan or not)
- extra dried and fresh Blueberries
- Coconut Milk

Method

Pre heat oven to 350 degrees F with the rack in the center. Lightly coat a 13X9X2" inch baking dish with cooking spray. Combine all ingredients in a large bowl adding blueberries and coconut last. Sweeten to taste (I used 2 droppers full of vanilla stevia drops.) Bake for about one hour. The oatmeal will appear not done when you take it out of the oven. Remove from the oven and let it cool to room temperature. Then put it in your refrigerator overnight for best results. It will thicken nicely in there.

Heat the blueberries with a splash of water over medium high heat. When you hear them sizzle reduce heat to medium and cook for about 5 minutes until saucy. Mash the blueberries against the side of the pan with a spatula. Serve oatmeal with some almond or coconut milk and blueberry sauce.

Cook this oatmeal the night before you plan on serving it so I has time to thicken in the refrigerator.

Re-heat portions before serving

Blueberry Almond (Date-Sweetened) Muffins Recipe

Makes **6** muffins

Ingredients
- 1 cup brown rice flour
- 1/2 tsp baking soda
- 1 tsp baking powder
- 1/4 tsp salt
- 7-8 large dried dates
- ~ 1/2 cup almond or soy milk*
- 1 1/2 TB flax seeds, coarsely ground
- 1 TB lemon juice & 1-2 tsp zest
- 1/3 cup applesauce
- 1/2 tsp vanilla extract
- 1/2 cup fresh blueberries
- 1/4 cup sliced almonds, toasted

1. Preheat oven to 400 degrees. Prepare a muffin pan with liners. Place the dates in a small blender or processor. Pulse until the dates are finely chopped. Add the applesauce to the dates and process or blend until the mixture turns into a smooth paste.

2. Combine all of the wet ingrdients: mixture from step 1, almond/soy milk, lemon juice + zest, and vanilla extract. Add the ground seed to the wet ingredients. Mix well. Set aside.

3. Whisk together brown rice flour, baking soda, baking powder, and salt. Add the wet ingredients from step two to the dry ingredients. Mix until the ingredients are just combined. Add the blueberries and almond slices. Stir gently. Using a ice cream or batter scoop, divide the batter into 6 muffins cups/liners. If you'd like, you can sprinkle some raw almond slices on top.

4. Bake on the center rack for 22-25 minutes until a toothpick comes out clean. Rotate the muffin pan midway to ensure even baking. Remove from oven and allow the muffins to cool in the muffin tin

for about 10-15 minutes. Transfer to a cooling rack and allow the muffins to cool completely.

The muffins are yummier when they are allowed to cool completely. Once cooled, you can really taste the sweetness from the dates. They actually taste better the morning after! So enjoy them for breakfast the next day or as a tasty snack. They make great healthy snacks for kids too!

Banana-Apple Buckwheat Muffins

Ingredients

- 1/4 cup buckwheat flour
- 1 tsp baking powder
- 1/2 tsp ground cinnamon
- 1/8 tsp coarse salt
- 2 large eggs
- 1/2 mashed banana
- 1/4 cup honey
- 1/2 finely diced (peeled and cored) sweet apple (such as Honeycrisp)
- 1/4 cup chopped walnuts

Directions

1. Heat oven to 350 degrees. Place four baking cups in a muffin tin.
2. In a bowl, whisk together flour, baking powder, cinnamon, and salt. In another bowl, whisk together eggs, banana, and honey. Mix the wet ingredients into the dry, then fold in apple and walnuts.
3. Fill the batter to the tops of the lined cups and fill remaining cups halfway with water.
4. Bake 30 minutes, or until a tester comes out clean. Let cool on a wire rack.
5. ENJOY.........

Veggie Quinoa Breakfast Bowl

yield: 1 serving

- 1/2 cup of quinoa, rinsed
- 1/2 cup of milk
- 1/2 cup of water
- broccoli, cut into florets
- mushrooms, sliced
- cheddar cheese, grated
- salt & pepper, to taste
- 1 egg

Heat a little bit of olive oil in a pan over medium high. Add broccoli and mushrooms, and stir-fry until cooked (around 5 minutes). Remove from heat and set aside. Combine milk, water, and quinoa in a large saucepan. Bring to a boil, then reduce heat to low. Simmer, stirring regularly*, until most of the liquid has been absorbed. Add vegetables, cheese, and salt & pepper to the pot of quinoa and stir to combine. Cover and set aside. Fry a sunny side–up egg. Transfer the quinoa to a bowl, then top with the egg. Enjoy..

Chia Seed Breakfast Bowl

Ingredients:

Chia mixture

- 4 tbsp chia seeds
- 1 – 1.25 cups almond milk (it's great made with Homemade Almond Milk)
- 2 small bananas, chopped small
- 1/2 tsp pure vanilla extract
- two pinches of cinnamon

Toppings:

- 2 tbsp raw buckwheat groats, soaked
- 2 tbsp raisins, soaked
- 2 tbsp whole raw almonds, chopped and soaked
- couples pinches of cinnamon
- 2 tbsp hemp seeds

1. Mash bananas in a medium-sized bowl. Stir in chia seeds. Whisk in the almond milk, vanilla, and cinnamon until combined. Place in fridge overnight to thicken.

2. Add buckwheat groats, raisins, and chopped almonds into another bowl. Cover in water and soak overnight in the fridge or on the counter.

3. In the morning, place your desired amount of chia pudding into a bowl. (Note: at this point, you can blend your chia pudding if a smooth texture is desired, but I don't bother). You can add more almond milk if you want to thin it out in the morning. Or, if it's too thin, add more chia seeds to thicken it up. Drain and rinse the buckwheat/almond/raisin mixture. Sprinkle on top of chia mixture along with a pinch of cinnamon and a tablespoon of hemp

seeds. Serve with a drizzle of maple syrup, if desired. Store leftovers in the fridge for 1-2 days.

Vanilla Chia Pudding

- 1 1/2 cups milk (I used whole milk, but you can use almond or soy or whatever you drink. No skim though)
- 1/4 cup chia seeds
- 1 tsp pure vanilla
- 1 tbsp maple syrup

Combine all ingredients in large bowl. Whisk well. Refrigerate and whisk every 10 minutes, for half hour. This is so it doesn't get lumpy. After half hour, pour into 4 serving dishes, cover and refrigerate for at least 3 hours. Garnish with fresh berries. Serves 4.

HONEY WHOLE GRAIN BREAD

1 1/2 cups warm water (100-110*F)
1 tsp cane sugar
1 package (2 1/4 tsp) active dry yeast
1/4 cup honey
2 tbsp extra virgin olive oil
1 tbsp apple cider vinegar
1/2 cup arrowroot powder
1/2 cup tapioca flour
1/2 cup brown rice flour
1/2 cup sorghum flour
1/2 cup teff flour
1/4 cup buckwheat flour
1/4 cup amaranth flour
1 1/2 tsp xanthan gum
1 tsp salt
1/2 tsp baking soda

Preheat oven to 200*F. Grease a 9x5 loaf pan with olive oil.
Place warm water, sugar and yeast in medium bowl and stir. Make sure
water is right temp - yeast should bubble up. If it doesn't, start over. Let it
stand, bubbling away for 5-10 minutes. Stir in honey, oil and vinegar. Whisk
well.
Combine dry ingredients in bowl of stand mixer. Pour in yeast mixture. Mix
on medium for about a minute. Pour into loaf pan. Place uncovered in
200*F oven, leaving door cracked open. Let it rise for 35 minutes. Close
door, increase heat to 375*F and bake for 30 minutes, or until toothpick
inserted comes out clean. Loosen from pan and place onto cooling rack.
Makes one loaf.

Charred Tomatoes with Fried Eggs on Garlic Toast

INGREDIENTS
- 4 slices rustic bread, toasted
- 1 clove garlic, peeled
- 1 tablespoon extra-virgin olive oil, plus more for brushing
- 4 large eggs
- Coarse salt and freshly ground pepper
- 4 small tomatoes, such as cocktail or Campari, halved

DIRECTIONS
1. STEP 1

Rub toasted bread with garlic and brush with oil. Heat oil in a large, heavy skillet (preferably cast-iron) over medium heat. Crack eggs into skillet and cook, undisturbed, until whites are set, 2 to 3 minutes. Season with salt and pepper and transfer to a plate.

2. STEP 2

Increase heat to medium-high. Brush cut sides of tomatoes with oil. Sear, cut sides down and undisturbed, until charred, 3 to 4 minutes. Transfer 2 tomato halves to each piece of toast with a spatula and lightly mash. Season with salt and pepper and top with fried eggs.

Baked Sweet Potato with Greens

Ingredients
- 2 pricked sweet potatoes
- 1 Tbsp extra-virgin olive oil
- 1 thinly sliced small onion
- 1 stemmed and chopped bunch Swiss chard
- Coarse salt
- 1 sliced avocado, divided
- Cayenne
- Lemon

Directions
1. Heat oven to 400 degrees. Bake sweet potatoes until tender, about 45 minutes.
2. Heat oil in a large skillet over medium heat. Add onion and cook until tender, about 6 minutes. Add chard and cook, stirring, until bright green and wilted, about 5 minutes. Season with salt.
3. To serve, split potatoes and top each with the greens and 1/2 sliced avocado. Season with cayenne, salt, and a squeeze of lemon.

Thai Curry with Tilapia and Veggies

Ingredients

- 1 tbsp coconut oil (or any cooking oil)
- 1 small red onion
- 1 bunch of green beans
- 1 large carrot
- 1 red pepper
- 1 can coconut milk
- 3 tbsp thai red curry paste
- 3 tilapia fillets
- diced cilantro
- 1 green onion
- lime
- pinch of salt

Instructions

1. Heat a large pan to medium heat.
2. Melt coconut oil in the pan, and saute onion until it starts to soften.
3. Add green beans and cook for about 5 minutes.
4. Add carrot and red pepper.
5. Add curry paste and coconut milk to the pan. Stir until the curry paste is fully dissolved into the coconut milk.
6. Cook for 5 minutes.
7. Add fish and cook for 5 to 6 minutes (until done).
8. Add salt to taste.
9. Serve on top of your favorite rice, millet, or quinoa.
10. Garnish with cilantro, green onion, and a wedge of lime.

Maple Roasted Chickpeas

Yields about 1 cup
- 15 ounce can (425 grams) canned chickpeas/garbanzo beans
- 2 teaspoons vegetable oil
- 1 teaspoon ground cinnamon
- 1 tablespoon brown sugar
- 1 tablespoon pure maple syrup

Method:
Preheat oven to 375 degrees F (190 degrees C).
Drain and rinse garbanzo beans, running them under cool water for several minutes to clean off the starch. You may optionally remove the skins from the beans (it does take a few minutes) or you can leave them on—it's your personal preference. Dry off the beans.
In a small bowl, whisk together the oil, cinnamon, and brown sugar. Place beans in bowl and stir until evenly coated. Spread out the beans on a large baking sheet and bake for 35-40 minutes, or until beans are crunchy and no longer soft in the middle. Test taste every few minutes until desired texture is reached.
Place hot, roasted beans in a small bowl and coat evenly with maple syrup. Spread beans back out on baking sheet and allow to dry. Store in an airtight container at room temperature.

Black Bean & Quinoa Veggie Burgers

- Patties:
  ½ cup dry quinoa
  1 tsp olive oil
  1/2 red onion, chopped
  3 cloves garlic, minced
  1/2 tsp Kosher salt, divided
  1 (15 oz) can black beans, drained and rinsed
  2 Tbsp tomato paste
  1 large egg
  2/3 cup frozen corn
  1/2 cup cilantro, chopped
  1 chipotle in adobo, minced
  2 tsp ground cumin
  1/2 cup rolled oats
  1/4 cup oat flour

- Yogurt Sauce:
  ½ cup plain fat-free Greek yogurt
  1 Tbsp honey
  1 Tbsp Dijon mustard

Directions:
Place the quinoa in a small saucepan with 1 cup of water. Set the saucepan over medium-high heat and bring to a boil. Reduce heat to low, cover the pan, and cook 10-15 minutes until the water is absorbed and quinoa is cooked. Remove from heat. Note: this step can be done ahead of time. Heat the oil in a small pan over medium heat and add the onion and garlic. Add 1/4 teaspoon salt and sauté until onions are softened, 5-6 minutes. Place the mixture into a large bowl. Add black beans to the bowl and using a potato masher or fork, mash together until a pasty mixture forms.

Stir in the tomato paste, egg, corn, cilantro, chipotles, cumin and remaining 1/4 teaspoon salt. Stir in the cooked quinoa, oats, and oat flour until well mixed. Form the mixture into 6 equal patties, compacting them well with your hands as you form them. Place the patties on a baking sheet, cover them with plastic wrap and refrigerate for at least a few hours or overnight. To make the yogurt sauce, stir the yogurt, honey and mustard together in a small bowl.

When ready to eat, preheat the oven to 400 F or heat a griddle to medium-high heat. If baking, spray a baking sheet with nonstick cooking spray and place the patties on the sheet cook 10-12 minutes until the patties are golden brown and crispy. Carefully flip the over and cook another 10 minutes. If using a griddle, heat 4-6 minutes per side or until slightly golden. Serve patties with the yogurt sauce.

Savory Pumpkin/Flaxseed Onion Crackers

Ingredients
- 1 c Flax seed
- 1 c Water
- 1 heaping Tbsp Date Paste
- 4 cups Pumpkin Seeds
- 4 cups chopped Pumpkin seeds
- 1/2 c chopped Green Onion (or onion of choice)
- 2 Tbsp Onion powder
- 1/2 tsp Black Pepper
- 1.5 tsp Salt

Methods/steps
1) In a bowl combine together your flax seeds and water. Let soak for 1 hour until it become thick and gelatinous. No, really, this is what we want!
2) Mix date paste into your gelatinous soaked Flaxseeds. Set this mixture aside for later.
3) In your food processor (or using one of the methods noted before the recipe) proceed to pulse/grind your pumpkin seeds. The goal is to roughly chop them up, but not grind them into a powder.
4) In a large mixing bowl combine your crushed pumpkin seeds with your chopped green onion, onion powder, black pepper and salt. Mix well. Create a well in your ingredients and proceed to add the Flax/Water/Date mixture that you'd set aside.
5) Mix everything together. At this point you will have a crumbly wet Cracker mixture, this is great!

Final Step: Assembling and Drying
1) Use a fork or small spatula to gently press, shape and flatten out your cracker mixture to roughly 1/4" thickness on a sheet of parchment paper or teflon sheet.
Helpful Hint: I recommend having a small cup of water at your station and lightly dampening your fork or spatula as you flatten out/shape your crackers. This helps immensely, as the cracker batter tends to be sticky. Don't worry, the additional water from the fork/spatula won't alter the crackers texture.
2) Score your crackers into desired dimensions before you move on to drying them

Eggplant Pesto

Ingredients
- 1 medium eggplant
- 1/4 cup blanched almond slivers, soaked in water
- 3-4 sun dried tomatoes (not the ones packaged in oil)
- 2-3 cup basil leaves, depending on how strong you like the basil flavor to be
- 2 cloves garlic
- 2 tsp. cilantro or parsley
- Optional: Almond milk as needed to make the sauce more liquid

1. Before you begin, soak the almond slivers in water for at least 2 hours.
2. Slice up the eggplant, drizzle it with a little bit of olive oil and roast it for about 30 minutes at 450. You want it to be mushy but cooked enough to take away the bitterness.
3. Once roasted, remove eggplant from oven and blend everything together in a food processor. That's it! If you want a liquid-y consistency, just add some almond (or other non-dairy) milk.

Cinnamon Fruit Kebobs

Ingredients:
- 1 fresh, ripe pineapple
- 6 white nectarines
- 6 plums
- Juice from the fruit
- 1 tablespoon honey
- 1 teaspoon cinnamon

Directions:
1. Cut all your fruits into bite-sized chunks. Be sure to cut them over a large bowl (the bowl that holds the fruit before you skewer it). You want to save as much of the juice as possible for the basting sauce.
2. Add the honey and cinnamon to the juice and mix well. This is your basting sauce.
3. Put the fruit chunks on skewers.
4. Put the kebobs on the BBQ and, using a basting brush, baste the kebobs with the basting sauce.
5. The kebobs are done when they have a nice golden brown color. I BBQ'd mine for approximately 30 minutes. But use your judgment. The fruit should be nice and caramelized.

Roasted Sweet Potato Salad

Ingredients:

- 1/2 lb. (227 g) peeled sweet potatoes, cut into small cubes
- 2 small red onions, cut into quarters or eighths
- 3 tbsp. olive oil
- 1 head garlic, top cut off for roasting
- 2 tsp. fresh thyme, chopped
- 1/2 tsp. balsamic vinegar
- Sea salt to taste

Directions:

1. Preheat oven to 350 F.
2. Place the cut potatoes in a plastic bag with the oil. Shake well to coat and pour out onto an ungreased cookie sheet, but don't pour out all the oil yet.
3. Put the onions in the same bag and toss that to coat with oil as well. Toss the onions and potatoes separately because you will be chopping the onions later.
4. Set the head of garlic on the pan for roasting as well.
5. Pour the onions out onto the same cookie sheet along with any remaining oil.
6. Spread out so the vegetables are in a single layer.
7. Roast the vegetables for approximately 45 minutes, or until they are soft and cooked through and the potatoes are slightly golden edges. The garlic should have one or two cloves popping out to let you know it's done.
8. Allow to cool a bit. Then squeeze the garlic out of the head.
9. Cut the onions down to small pieces and toss all ingredients together in a mixing bowl.
10. Serve as a side dish.

Cinnamon Apple Bread

Ingredients:
- 2 cups whole wheat pastry flour
- 1 cup sucanat
- 1 teaspoon cinnamon
- 1/4 cup oil (light flavored oil like grape seed or safflower)
- 1/4 cup unsweetened apple sauce
- 4 medium cooking apples, peeled, cored and chopped fine
- 1 large egg, beaten
- Dulce De Leche for topping (Trust me, you want the topping on this.)

Directions:
1. Preheat to 350.
2. In a large mixing bowl, whisk together the flour, sucanat and cinnamon.
3. Stir in the oil, apple sauce, apples and egg.
4. Mix well.
5. Scrape into a 9X13 baking dish and bake for 1 to 1 1/2 hours or until a knife inserted into the middle pulls out clean.

Freedom Brownies

Ingredients:
- 1/3 cup coconut flour
- 1/3 cup unsweetened cocoa powder
- 1/3 cup coconut oil
- 5 whole eggs
- 1/2 cup maple syrup
- 2 teaspoons pure vanilla extract, no sugar added

Directions:
1. In a medium mixing bowl, whisk together the coconut flour and cocoa powder.
2. Whisk in the coconut oil, eggs, maple syrup and vanilla extract. Blend well.
3. Pour batter into a greased baking dish (mine was about 7×11), and bake at 350 F. for about 30 minutes.
4. Allow to cool. This is important because they tend to fall apart easily when warm, making it difficult to get them out of the pan.

Coconut Lime Freezer Cookies

Ingredients:
- 1/4 cup honey
- 1 teaspoon vanilla
- 1/4 cup creamy peanut butter
- 2 tablespoon psyllium husks (you can substitute with wheat germ or oat bran too.)
- 1/2 cup quick-cooking oats
- 2 tablespoon dried coconut
- Zest of 1 lime
- Juice of 1 lime

Directions:
1. Mix all ingredients together thoroughly in a medium mixing bowl.
2. Spoon dough out onto a parchment lined cookie sheet in 12 equal portions (just slightly smaller than walnut size)
3. Place in freezer for at least 2 hours and serve.

BBQ Carrots

Ingredients:
- 2 pounds organic baby carrots
- 1 teaspoon black pepper
- 1 tablespoon onion powder
- 1 tablespoon garlic powder
- 1 tablespoon olive oil

Directions:
1. Place all ingredients inside a large plastic bag, seal and shake until the carrots are well coated.
2. Place a piece of aluminum foil on the BBQ grill and place your carrots on that. Spread them out so that they are in a single layer.
3. Put the lid on the grill and allow to cook for about 30 minutes, stirring occasionally with BBQ tongs. Cook until they are soft and easily pierced with a fork.

Note: Cooking times will vary based on the temperature of your grill. 30 minutes is an approximate time.

Caution: These little buggers really hold their heat! Cutting them and allowing them to cool for a bit before eating them is probably a wise decision.

Cilantro Salsa

Ingredients:
- 5-6 small-medium tomatoes
- 4 small garlic cloves (or two large ones)
- Jalapeño peppers (choose the type & amount based on how spicy you like your salsa)
- Cilantro (about 1/2 cup chopped, but again, use to your liking)
- Red onion (1 large or two small)

Directions:
1. Chop all your ingredients. Be sure you chop them well. The finer you chop everything, the better texture your salsa will have.
2. Mix in a bowl and serve.

Snickerdoodles

(Yield: 10 cookies)

Ingredients:

- 3/4 Cup (100g) almond flour (ground almonds)
- 1/4 teaspoon baking soda
- 1/2 teaspoon ground cinnamon
- 1 tablespoon pure maple syrup
- 2 tablespoons smooth cashew nut butter
- 2 tablespoons almond milk
- 1 teaspoon pure vanilla extract
- **For the topping:**
- 1/2 tablespoon coconut sugar
- 1/4 teaspoon ground cinnamon

Directions:

1. Preheat the oven to 350F and line a cookie sheet with some baking parchment
2. Place the topping ingredients into a bowl and set aside
3. Place the almond flour, baking soda and cinnamon into a mixing bowl and stir to combine.
4. Add the maple syrup, cashew nut butter, almond milk and vanilla and give the whole thing a mix until thoroughly combined. (The dough will seem quite wet and sticky)
5. Take out 1 Tablespoon of the mixture and with clean, dry hands roll the dough into a ball and place onto the parchment paper. (I washed and dried my hands in between each one)
6. Repeat this process until you have used up all of the mixture. It should make around 10 cookies.
7. Once you have the cookie balls ready, gently press each one down into a 'cookie' shape with your first two fingers. A little raised in the centre and slightly flatter around the edges. (The cookies won't change shape much in the oven at all so this is the time to make them pretty!).
8. Give the topping mixture you prepared earlier a little mix, and sprinkle it over the top of the cookies, gently rubbing it with your fingers to make it stick.
9. Carefully shake off any excess topping mixture from the pan and then place the cookie sheet into the oven for 10 – 15 minutes. (Mine cooked in 12 minutes)
10. Once golden brown, remove from the oven and place onto a wire rack to cool a little before serving.

Italian Herb BBQ Crookneck Squash

Ingredients:
- 2 pounds crookneck (yellow) squash
- 1 tablespoon olive oil
- 1 tablespoon italian seasoning
- 1 tablespoon garlic powder
- 2 teaspoons onion powder
- Parmesan cheese for garnish (optional)

\Directions:
1. In a large, food-safe bag, combine all ingredients and shake well to coat evenly.
2. Pour into a BBQ pan and grill until soft.
3. Top with parmesan if you wish and serve.

Note: If you don't have a barbecue pan, you can cook this on the stovetop as well. Simply sauté everything together over low to medium heat and enjoy.

Rosemary Sweet Potatoes

Ingredients:
- 2 medium sweet potatoes, washed and sliced (peel if preferred)
- 1 tablespoon olive oil
- 2 tablespoons fresh, chopped rosemary
- 1 teaspoon garlic powder

Directions:
1. Peel (if desired) and slice your sweet potatoes very thin. About 1/8 to 1/4 inch thick at the most. The thinner they are, the better they cook.
2. Place all ingredients in a large, food-safe bag and shake to coat the potatoes in the oil and spices.
3. Using a grill pan or aluminum foil, cook the potatoes on the grill. They may take a while to cook, so allow for that. They will take a bit longer to cook than most pieces of meat. So time your meal accordingly. They are done with they begin to fall apart when stirred.

BBQ Zucchini

Ingredients:
- 2 pounds zucchini, quartered
- 2 tablespoons garlic powder
- 2 tablespoons onion powder
- 1/4 teaspoon salt
- 1/2 teaspoon black pepper
- 1/4 cup olive oil

Directions:
1. Place all ingredients into a plastic bag, and gently shake until the zucchini is coated in the oil and spices.
2. Place on BBQ and cook. (Much of the oil will be left behind in the bag. That's okay. I just toss it with the bag.)
3. When the zucchini is cooked to your liking, remove from the grill and allow to cool. These retain A LOT of heat. So cooling time is essential.

NOTE: For crispier/crunchier zucchini, cook on higher heat for a shorter time. For a softer zucchini, cook on lower heat for a longer time.

Lemon Portobello Mushroom Burgers

Ingredients:
- 4 Large portobello mushrooms
- 2 tablespoons olive oil
- 1 tablespoon garlic powder
- 1 tablespoon onion powder
- 1/2 cup lemon juice
- Zest of 1 lemon

Directions:
1. Place all ingredients in a disposable plastic bag and gently move everything around in the bag so the seasoning gets evenly distributed over the mushrooms.
2. Place on the bbq and cook until the mushrooms are very soft and easily sliced.
3. Assemble your burger to your liking. That's it!